Your Drugs & Sex

How Prescription & Non-Prescription Drugs Can Affect Your Sex Life

P. J. Bush, PhD
R. B. Raffa, PhD
A. I. Wertheimer, PhD

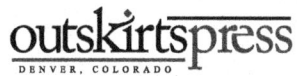

The opinions expressed in this manuscript are solely the opinions of the authors and do not represent the opinions or thoughts of the publisher. The authors have represented and warranted full ownership and/or legal right to publish all the materials in this book.

Your Drugs and Sex
How Prescription & Non-Prescription Drugs Can Affect Your Sex Life
All Rights Reserved.
Copyright © 2015 P.J. Bush, R.B. Raffa, A.I. Wertheimer
4.0

The cover images were purchased from Dreamstime.com.

This book may not be reproduced, transmitted, or stored in whole or in part by any means, including graphic, electronic, or mechanical without the express written consent of the publisher except in the case of brief quotations embodied in critical articles and reviews.

Outskirts Press, Inc.
http://www.outskirtspress.com

ISBN: 978-1-4787-3840-4

Outskirts Press and the "OP" logo are trademarks belonging to Outskirts Press, Inc.

PRINTED IN THE UNITED STATES OF AMERICA

Contents

About the Authors i
Disclaimers iii
Preface v
Navigating This Book vii
A Note About Sexual Arousal and Performance ix

Part One: Male and Female Sexual Anatomy & Physiology 1
1. Male Sexual Anatomy & Physiology 3
2. Female Sexual Anatomy & Physiology 8

Part Two: Most Frequently Prescribed Meds: Which Affect Sex Performance? ... 13
3. Medicines Can Affect Your Sex Life 15
4. Is Your Med on This List 21

Part Three: Meds Used to Improve Sex 25
5. Male Performance Enhancers 27
6. Female Performance Enhancers 38
7. Aphrodiasics and Placebos 47

Part Four: Contraception 51
8. The Pill and Other Female Contraceptives: Can They Affect Your Sex Life? 53

Part Five: Prescription Meds 63
9. Blood Pressure Meds 65

10. Cholesterol Lowering Meds 75
11. Antidepressants 79
12. Minor Tranquilizers and Anti-Anxiety Meds 87
13. Antipsychotics 90
14. And a Few Others 95

Part Six: Nonmedical Med Use *97*
15. Legal Meds Used for Nonmedical Purposes:
    Can They Affect Your Sex Life? 99

Part Seven: Over-the-Counter Meds *121*
16. Over-the-Counter and into the Bedroom 123

Part Eight: What You Can Do *129*
17. Getting Help from Your Doctor or Pharmacist 131
18. Good Medical Information Sources 134

Appendices *141*
Appendix A: Most Frequently Prescribed Drugs and Sex Effects 143
Appendix B: References 151

About the Authors

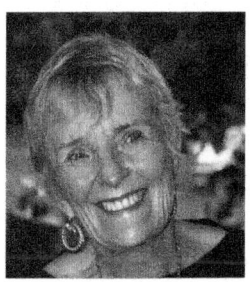

Patricia J. Bush, PhD

Dr. Bush is emeritus professor at Georgetown University School of Medicine, where she chaired the Division of Children's Health Promotion in the Department of Family Medicine. She earned a B.S. in Pharmacy from the University of Michigan, an M.Sc. in medical sociology at the University of London (UK), and a PhD in social pharmacy at the University of Minnesota. She has been the recipient of numerous research grants, and has published 8 books, 21 book chapters and more than 110 articles in peer-reviewed journals. She has been a consultant to a number of organizations, including the U.S. Pharmacopeia. Her areas of expertise include medicine use behaviors, and she is most well known for her studies in children's medicine knowledge, attitudes and behaviors.

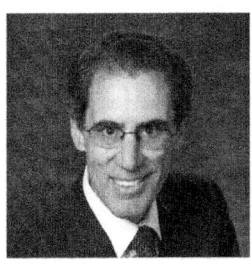

Robert B. Raffa, PhD

Dr. Raffa is Professor of Pharmacology in the Department of Pharmaceutical Sciences at Temple University School of Pharmacy and Research Professor in the Department of Pharmacology of Temple University's School of Medicine. He holds bachelor's degrees in Chemical Engineering and Physiological Psychology from the University of Delaware, master's degrees in Biomedical Engineering (Drexel University) and Toxicology (Thomas Jefferson University). Dr. Raffa holds a PhD in Pharmacology from Temple University. He was a research Fellow and co-leader for analgesics discovery at Johnson and Johnson. He is the holder of several patents and he has published over 270 papers in refereed journals, is the co-author of several books, and the co-editor of the Journal of Clinical Pharmacy and Therapeutics.

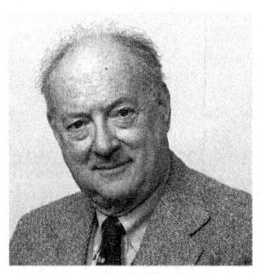

Albert I Wertheimer, PhD

Dr. Wertheimer is Professor of Pharmacy Administration in the Department of Pharmacy Practice at Temple University School of Pharmacy in Philadelphia. He is the editor of the Journal of Pharmaceutical Health Services Research, and is an international authority in pharmacoeconomics and outcomes research. He was the recipient of the FIP 2008 Andre Bedat Award for outstanding contributions to international pharmacy. He earned a Pharmacy degree at the University of Buffalo, an MBA from the State University of New York at Buffalo and a PhD degree from Purdue University. He has published 34 books and over 400 journal articles.

Disclaimers

This book contains information obtained from authentic and highly regarded sources. Reasonable efforts have been made to publish reliable data and information, however the authors and publisher cannot assume responsibility for the validity of all materials or the consequence of their use. The authors and publisher have attempted to trace the copyright holders of all material reproduced in this publication and apologize to any copyright holders if permission to publish in this form has not been obtained. If any copyright material has not been properly acknowledged, please write and let us know so we may rectify in any future reprint.

Preface

Maybe your sex life isn't what it used to be. Maybe it isn't even what you think or hoped that it would be at your age. Or perhaps you have disappointed your sexual partner on more than one occasion by not being able to perform sexually as hoped or expected by you or by them. "What's wrong?" you–or they–might ask.

Good question. What IS wrong? Perhaps it is just the situation. You just might not be in the mood, or it's not the right time or place, or maybe not the right person. Or maybe you are anxious. Anxious about getting caught, or getting a sexually-transmitted disease, or getting pregnant, or breaking a religious taboo or prohibition. Or maybe you are worried about your job(s), your finances, or your health; or maybe you have problems with your teenage children, siblings, elderly parents, neighbors, the IRS, or those little voices that you keep hearing in your head. Or perhaps you are just angry at your partner right now because your partner forgot it was your birthday, or wedding anniversary! Luckily, none of these problems are medical (even though they do of course involve physiology and biochemistry at some level). They will most likely disappear and blissfully be forgotten as soon as the situation is resolved. It was only temporary. Joy (= sex) will return and life will be good again.

But perhaps it is not the situation, the other person, or something else. Perhaps it seems to be YOU! What is happening? This is not typical for you. You were always pretty good in sexual performance. Could it be increasing age? Could it be something medical? The answer to both of these questions is: yes, it possibly might be. A quick trip to the doctor for a check-up will help determine if this is really the case. But there is another possibility that you might not be aware of. The cause could be a medicine that you are taking ... and that is the subject of this book.

This book is intended for the average person. It is for someone who is taking, or is thinking of taking, a medicine or other substance (such as herbal or even abused drug) intended to produce an effect on the body. The medicine could be one that requires a prescription (from a doctor) or does not (nonprescription; available at a pharmacy). We start with the very basics, which can be skipped if not needed, and progress to more scientific if wanted (including a few references as a guide to additional information). Our primary goal was that this book is helpful to everyone.

We wish to acknowledge and thank many people who played a role in this book: our families and others who encouraged us, in the past and recently; and those who read early versions and gave helpful advice, particularly Joaquima Serradell, PhD and Frank Breve, PharmD.

Navigating This Book

Suggestions on how to get the most out of this book from its authors

We envisioned readers using this book in two different ways. There is no "correct" way, so any way you want to dive into it is OK. However, let us suggest two paths for your consideration. If your immediate interest is to learn whether any of the medicines you are using or considering using might affect your sexual performance, we suggest going directly to Appendix A, a summary table of drugs and sex, to look up the medicines you are wondering about. Right there, if you see a page number after your drug, you can go there to learn more about the possible impact of that drug on your sex life. If no page number is there, it means that the authors found no reports in the scientific literature regarding any sex issues with that drug. We have listed the most widely prescribed drugs in the United States, which account for about 85% of all prescriptions. There are tens of thousands of other prescription drugs on the market in the United States, but reviewing all of them would not have been practical. Also the book does not focus on over-the-counter drugs; however, Chapter 16 is about those that might affect your sex life.

The other way we suggest using this book is to pick out specific chapters and read them when you feel like it. If you find that one or more of your meds is implicated with possible sexual performance issues, either to harm or help them, you might want to follow some of the suggested sources for additional information, possibly to find examples of other meds that might help you, and possibly to discuss what you have learned with your physician at your next visit.

And last, a few words of caution. This book is no substitute for your physician. Sexual performance is influenced by many factors besides medicines. Depression, diabetes, high blood pressure, and other conditions influence sexual performance as does advancing age. We urge you to be open and initiate a conversation with your physician if you are not satisfied with your sexual performance. Don't be ashamed. You are not the first person your physician has had this conversation with. As you will see in the following chapters, in addition to learning what meds to possibly avoid, there is plenty of information about meds and products your physician can suggest or prescribe to improve your sex life.

A Note About Sexual Arousal and Performance

What is considered a 'disorder' in sexual arousal or performance? First of all, it is very important to recognize that the timing, extent, and appropriateness of the expression of sexual activity are a matter of personal choice, and that they depend to a large extent on the maturity, age, cultural, and other factors that influence the person and how they view sexual behavior.

A person might desire to engage in sexual activities considered abnormally high in relation to normal development or cultural norms. If this is a reasoned and free choice, it is not a disorder. On the other hand, they might have a physical condition that is a disorder, such as genital-arousal disorder (an uncontrollable and persistent sexual arousal). Thus 'hypersexual' activity can either be normal for that person or it be a sign of a physical or psychological disorder in another person.

Likewise, when a person fails to be aroused or to perform sexually in a situation that would normally produce such responses, it might be only temporary or it might be due to some physical or psychological impediment. It is important to note here, though, that everyone experiences some situations in which, for some reason, sexual arousal or performance just does not occur. Such occurrences – if they do not occur too frequently or can be explained by other reasons (e.g., too tired from physical exertion, worry over financial or other concerns, distraction, guilt, and many other possibilities) – are usually not signs of a disorder. But if the lack of arousal or sexual performance persists without other explanations, it might be a sign of a sexual arousal or performance disorder.

Some medications can produce changes in sexual arousal or performance. This is the topic of this book.

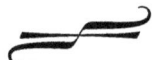

Part One
Male and Female
Sexual Anatomy & Physiology

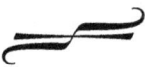

1

Male Sexual Anatomy & Physiology

"Of course, if I am nothing but an ego, and woman is nothing but another ego, then there is really no vital difference between us. Two little dolls of conscious entities, squeaking when you squeeze them. And with a tiny bit of an extraneous appendage to mark which is which..."

– D.H. Lawrence

Normal Male Sexual Anatomy

The organs of the male reproductive system produce, maintain, and transport sperm (the male reproductive cells) and semen (a protective fluid).[1]

Penis: The external male sex organ.[2] It has three major parts: the root (the part attached to the wall of the abdomen); a tubular body (shaft); and the glans (the cone-shaped end, also called the head). The glans is covered with a loose layer of skin (foreskin) unless removed (circumcision). Semen is transported to the end of the penis through the urethra.[3] The penis also contains sensitive nerve endings. The body of the penis contains chambers that are made up of sponge-like tissue that fill with blood when the male is sexually aroused. As it fills with blood, the penis becomes rigid and erect (an erection).[4] The skin of the penis is sufficiently loose and elastic to accommodate the change in penis size. During an erection, the flow of urine is normally blocked from the urethra, allowing only semen to be expelled (ejaculated) through the end of the penis when the male reaches sexual climax (orgasm).[5]

Scrotum: The loose pouch-like sac of skin that hangs behind and below the penis. Special muscles in the wall of the scrotum allow it to contract and relax in order to maintain the testicles (testes) at a temperature slightly cooler than the body temperature for normal sperm development. Moving the testicles closer to the body warms them; moving them farther away cools them.[6]

Testicles (testes): The oval organs responsible for making testosterone (the primary male sex hormone) and generating sperm lie in the scrotum and are attached at either end by the spermatic cord. Most men have two testes. Coiled tubes (seminiferous tubules) located within the testicles produce the sperm. [7]

Epididymis: A long, coiled tube within each testicle that transports and stores sperm cells while they mature (the sperm from the testicles are immature and are incapable of fertilization). During sexual arousal, contractions force the sperm out of the epididymis and into the vas deferens.

Vas deferens: The long, muscular tube that transports mature sperm to the urethra, the tube that carries sperm in preparation for ejaculation.[8]

Urethra: The tube from which semen is ejaculated. (It also carries urine from the bladder during urination, but the flow of urine is blocked from the urethra when the penis is erect, allowing only semen to be ejaculated at orgasm).

Seminal vesicles: Sac-like pouches attached to the vas deferens near the base of the bladder that produce a sugar-rich fluid that provides a source of energy for sperm to move (motility). This fluid makes up most of the volume of the ejaculate.[9]

Prostate gland: A walnut-sized structure located below the urinary bladder that contributes nourishing fluid to the ejaculate. The urethra, which carries the ejaculate that is expelled during orgasm, runs through the center of the prostate gland.[10]

Cowper's glands: Pea-sized structures located on the sides of the urethra just below the prostate gland that produce a clear, slippery fluid that empties into the urethra and serves to lubricate it and to neutralize any acidity that may be present due to residual drops of urine.

Normal Male Sexual Physiology

The male reproductive system is controlled by hormones, which are chemicals that regulate the activity of many different types of cells or organs.[11] The major hormones that are involved in the male reproductive system are gonadotropin-releasing hormone (GnRH), follicle-stimulating hormone (FSH), luteinizing hormone (LH), and testosterone. Females also have GnRH, FSH, LH, and testosterone (less than males).

GnRH is a hormone that is made and released from the hypothalamus[12] (which is an almond-size structure in the brain) that stimulates the pituitary gland (a pea-sized structure that extends from the base of the brain) to make and release FSH and LH.

FSH and **LH** are two hormones that are made and released from the pituitary gland that help regulate and time the development, pubertal maturation, and reproductive processes of the body.[13,14] They stimulate the production of sperm (spermatogenesis) by the testicles. They also work synergistically to stimulate the production of testosterone.

Testosterone is an androgen that plays a key role in the development of male characteristics, including muscle mass and strength, fat distribution, bone mass, facial hair growth, voice change, and sex drive. Testosterone levels follow a daily rhythm, which peaks early each day. Many other physiological, psychological, sociological, and environmental factors also affect testosterone levels.

Normal Male Sexual Arousal

Sexual arousal occurs when a male is exposed to physical or psychological (e.g., thoughts, pictures, or actions of others) stimulation, or even during sleep.[15-18] The sensitive nerve endings on the penis, together with nerve signals from the brain lead to widening of the blood vessels (vasodilation) in the penis and increased blood flow into the three spongy areas that run along the length of the shaft of the penis. As a result of the increase in the volume of blood entering the spongy regions of the penis, it enlarges and grows firm. At the same time, the skin of the scrotum is pulled tighter and the testicles are pulled up against the body.

As sexual arousal and stimulation continue, the glans or head of the erect penis will usually swell wider and deepen in color. The testicles can grow up to 50% larger as the genitals become filled with blood. With further sexual stimulation, the heart rate increases, blood pressure rises, and breathing quickens (hence, the caution that appears in the advertisements for some medications that a doctor's advice be sought before engaging in strenuous sexual activity).

As sexual arousal and stimulation continue further, the coordinated activity of muscles, the vas deferens, the seminal vesicles, and the prostate gland work to push sperm and semen into the part of the urethra inside the penis. [19] This marks the onset of orgasm and normally the man will continue to ejaculate even in the absence of continued stimulation. Repeated or prolonged stimulation without ejaculation can produce discomfort or even pain in the testicles — a condition that in every-day language is often called 'blue balls'.

If sexual arousal and stimulation cease before the male begins ejaculation, the process reverses. The blood leaves the spongy portions of the penis and returns to the rest of the body, the penis size reduces and other physical signs subside in a short time. Likewise, men usually experience a 'refractory period' following ejaculation. This is normal, and is characterized by loss of erection, reduced interest in immediate sex, and a feeling of relaxation. In physiological terms, this can be attributed to an increase in the levels of the neurohormones oxytocin (the 'love' hormone) and prolactin (sexual 'gratification'). How long the refractory period lasts is quite variable. It can be very short in an aroused young man or as long as a few hours or days in mid-life and older men. It also depends on the medical health of the man and the complex and wide range of psychological factors that increase or decrease sexual arousal.

The cognitive aspects of sexual arousal in men are not completely known, but they do involve the appraisal and evaluation of the stimulus, categorization of the stimulus as sexual, and an affective response.[20,21] Research suggests that cognitive factors, such as sexual motivation, perceived gender role expectations, and sexual attitudes, contribute to sex differences observed in subjective sexual arousal.[22] Specifically, while watching visual stimuli, men are more influenced by the sex of an actor portrayed in the stimulus, and men typically prefer a stimulus that allows objectification of the actor and projection of themselves into the scenario. There are reported differences in brain activation to sexual stimuli,[23] with men showing higher levels of amygdala and hypothalamus responses than women. This suggests the amygdala plays a critical role in the processing of sexually arousing visual stimuli in men.[20]

2

Female Sexual Anatomy & Physiology

"In youth, it was a way I had,
To do my best to please.
And change, with every passing lad
To suit his theories.

But now I know the things I know
And do the things I do,
And if you do not like me so,
To hell, my love, with you."

– Dorothy Parker,
The Complete Poems of Dorothy Parker

Female Sexual Anatomy

Vulva: The vulva includes all of a woman's external sex organs:[1,2]

Outer Lips: The outer lips are also called the labia majora, or outer labia. The outer lips are fleshy, covered by pubic hair, and connect to the thighs. Most women have larger outer lips than inner lips, but many women have larger inner lips than outer lips.

Inner Lips: The inner lips are also called the labia minora, or inner labia. They cover the vaginal opening and the urethra. Inner lips are visible when the outer labia are pulled apart. And in many women, the inner lips stick out of the outer lips. Inner lips can be short or long, wrinkled or smooth. The inner lips are also sensitive and can swell when a woman is aroused.[3] The inner lips can vary in color from pink to brownish black depending on the color of a woman's skin. The inner labia also can change color as women mature.

Clitoris[4-6]**:** The clitoris is the spongy tissue that fills with blood during sexual excitement and becomes erect. It is very sensitive to the touch. The external tip of the clitoris is located at the top of the vulva, where the inner lips meet. The inner structure of the clitoris includes a shaft and two crura — roots or legs — of erectile tissue that extend up to five inches into a woman's body on both sides of her vagina. Networks of highly sensitive nerves extend from the crura in the pelvic area. The clitoris is the only organ in the human body whose only purpose is sexual pleasure.

Clitoral Hood: The clitoral hood is the skin that covers and protects the external tip of the clitoris.

Opening of the Urethra: The urethra is the tube that empties the bladder and carries urine out of the body. The opening of the urethra is located below the clitoris. It is quite small and may be difficult to see or feel.

Opening of the Vagina: The vaginal opening is located below the urethral opening. The vaginal opening is where fingers, a penis, or tampons can enter the vagina and is also where menstrual blood and a fetus come out of the body.

Mons Veneris: The mons veneris is the fleshy, triangular mound above the vulva that is covered with pubic hair in adolescent and adult women. It cushions the pubic bone.

Vagina[7,8]**:** The vagina is the stretchable passage that connects a woman's external sex organs with her cervix and uterus.[9,10] The vagina is a tube with walls of wrinkled tissue that lay against one another. The walls open just enough to allow something to go in the vagina — like a tampon, finger, or penis.

The vagina is 2–4 inches long when a woman is not aroused and 4–8 inches long when she is sexually aroused. The vagina has three major functions:

- to allow menstrual flow to leave the body
- to allow sexual penetration to occur (either by hand, sex toy, or penis)
- to allow a fetus to pass through during vaginal delivery [11]

Cervix[12,13]**:** The cervix is the narrow, lower part of the uterus. It has an opening that connects the uterus to the vagina. This opening allows menstrual blood to leave the uterus and sperm to enter into the uterus, and is what dilates — stretches open — during labor.

Uterus[14]**:** The uterus is a pear-shaped, muscular reproductive organ from which women menstruate and where a normal pregnancy develops. The uterus is normally about the size of a woman's fist. It stretches many times that size during pregnancy. It is sometimes referred to as the womb.

During sexual arousal, the lower end of the uterus lifts toward the abdomen, which creates more space at the end of the vagina. This is called "tenting".

Fallopian Tubes: The fallopian tubes are two narrow tubes that carry eggs from the ovaries to the uterus. Sperm travels into the fallopian tubes to fertilize the egg.

Fimbriae: The fimbriae are like dozens of tiny fingers at the end of each fallopian tube that sweep the egg from the ovary into the tube.[15]

Ovaries: The ovaries are two organs that store eggs in a woman's body.[16] Ovaries also produce hormones, including estrogen, progesterone, and testosterone. During puberty, the ovaries start to release eggs each month and do so until menopause. Usually, one ovary releases an egg each month.

Bartholin's Glands: The Bartholin's glands are two glands that release fluid to lubricate the vagina during sexual arousal. They are located on either side of the vaginal opening.

Hymen: The hymen is the thin fleshy tissue that stretches across part of the opening to the vagina.[17,18]

G Spot: The G spot, or Gräfenberg spot, is located on the front wall of the vagina — the wall that is closest to the abdomen. It is about 1–2 inches inside the vagina.[19] The G spot is very sensitive and swells during sexual excitement.

Skene's Glands: The Skene's glands are located in the vulva on opposite sides of the opening to the urethra.[20] They release the fluid that is ejaculated during female ejaculation. They are also called paraurethral glands or female prostate glands.

Urethra: The urethra is the tube that empties the bladder and carries urine out of the body.

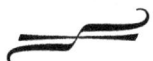

Part Two
Most Frequently Prescribed Meds: Which Affect Sex Performance?

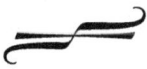

3

Medicines Can Affect Your Sex Life

"All substances are poisons; there is none which is not a poison. The right dose differentiates a poison from a remedy" [Sola dosis facit venenum]

— Paracelsus

There are many reasons that your sexual performance can be affected adversely; one of them is your medicine (prescription or nonprescription).[1-16] All medicines have some side effects (also called adverse effects). These side effects can appear in any system in the body, including systems that can affect sexual performance. And these don't have to be medicines taken for sexual purposes, they can be medicines taken for other conditions as well. For example, some commonly used medicines that have known sexual performance side effects include: lipid-lowering drugs such as the statins and fibrates (e.g., erectile dysfunction and, for both men and women, difficulty achieving orgasm); blood pressure lowering drugs such as the diuretics ("water pills"), beta-blockers, and alpha-blockers; antidepressant drugs (e.g., ejaculation failure, impotence, and decreased libido (sex drive)); antipsychotic medicines (estimated occurrence of 45 – 90%); anti-anxiety (anxiolytic) medicines (diminished orgasms, pain during intercourse, erectile dysfunction, and ejaculation problems); anti-ulcer (H-2 blocker) medicines (impotence); and anti-epileptic medicines (lower testosterone levels and cause erection problems for men, lubrication problems for women).

And there are others, as well. The good news is that in almost every case, there are alternative medicines or other options and for these, consult your doctor and pharmacist.

Increase in Medicine Use

The problem of sexual dysfunction caused by medicines is growing due to the large increase in the use of medicines. Advances in understanding the basic science of medical conditions such as high blood pressure, high levels of cholesterol (particularly LDL), diabetes, epilepsy, anxiety, depression, ADHD (attention deficit hyperactivity disorder), Parkinson's disease, and others have led to medicines that are now mainstays of medical care. Add to this the number of contraceptive medicines and OTC (over the counter) substances available for a host of less serious medical conditions or cosmetic purposes, and it is easy to see that the use of medicines is on the rise.

Percentage of persons using prescription drugs (number indicated) in the USA, 1988-2010

SOURCE: CDC/NCHS, Health, United States, 2013, Figure 20. Data from the National Health and Nutrition Examination Survey.

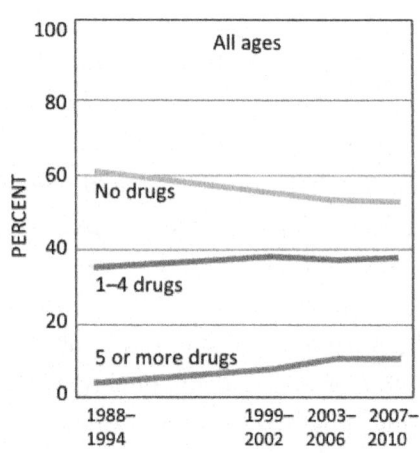

More Long-term Use

In addition to being prescribed more medicines, people are being prescribed them for longer periods of time. Back when the only truly effective medicines were the antibiotics, they were taken for only a short period of time (days or at most weeks). The same is true for most acute injuries: the pain reliever drug (analgesic) is taken until the injury heals. But what about medicines for diabetes, high blood pressure, epilepsy, high cholesterol, chronic pain, ADHD, Parkinson's disease, and one of these days Alzheimer's disease. The medicines currently available do not actually cure the problems, they only address the symptoms or other aspects of the problems. They must, therefore, be taken for long periods, perhaps for the remainder of one's life. Direct-to-consumer advertising and the ability to obtain prescription drugs *via* the Internet have also contributed to the increase in prescription and nonprescription drug use.

In addition to more medicines, for more diseases, and extended durations, people are living longer.[17] The life expectancy in the United States is about 50% longer now than it was in 1900. In 1900, the life expectancy for males was just a bit more than 40 years and for females it was just a bit over 48 years. At the end of the century, life expectancy for males was well over 70 years and for females it was just over 80 years. And as everyone knows, the older you get, the more medicines you usually need.

Use of Multiple Medicines

According to US government health statistics for the year 2007-2010, about ½ of all adults 20-59 years old had taken at least one prescription medicine and 7% had taken two. Almost ¼ of children 0-11 years old had taken at least one prescription medicine and 4.5% had taken two. The older population had even greater use. Almost 90% of all adults 60 and older had taken at least one prescription medicine, ¼ had taken 3-4 prescription medicines, and nearly 40% had taken a whopping five or more prescription medicines. And as the number of medicines you take increases, so do the side effects that might negatively affect sexual performance.

Prescription drug use in past month in USA by age, 2007-2010

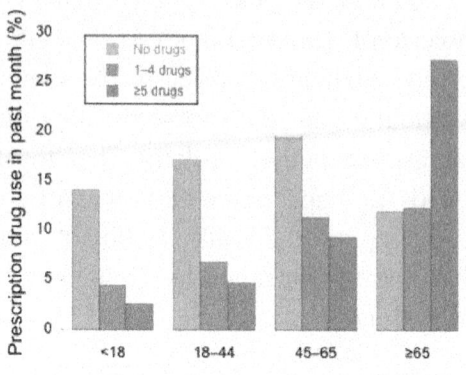

SOURCE: CDC/NCHS, Health, United States, 2013, Figure 20. Data from the National Health and Nutrition Examination Survey.

Category of prescription drugs used most often in USA, 1998–1994 vs 2007-2010

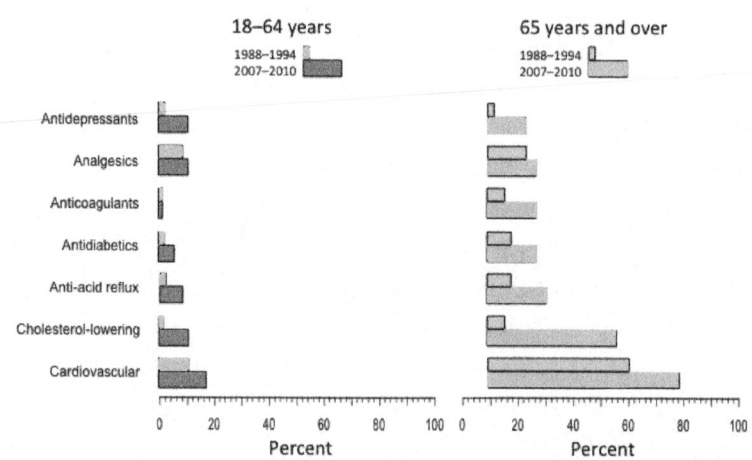

SOURCE: CDC/NCHS, Health, United States, 2013, Figure 21. Data from the National Health and Nutrition Examination Survey.

Increased Use of OTC Herbals, etc.

The use of plants and plant extracts for medicinal purposes dates from ancient times.[18-20] This is understandable, since plants have the ability to synthesize a wide variety of chemical compounds that are used in important biological functions within the plant and to defend it against attack from viruses, bacteria, and animals. In order to be effective against these threats, the chemicals must interact with the biochemistry of the attacker. As plants and animals co-evolved, some of the plant-derived chemicals became useful as a part of a mutually beneficial co-existence, and were co-opted for use by animals for their own biochemical processes. Thus, plant-derived compounds can produce their effects on the human body through processes that are similar to, or even identical to, the body's own. Some plant-sourced medicines include aspirin, codeine, digitalis, morphine, and quinine. Thus herbal medicines do not differ greatly from what we think of as modern medicines in terms of how they work. This enables herbal medicines to be as therapeutically effective as are prescription medicines (although it needs to be proven in each case by rigorous testing, just as in the case of prescription drugs).

But their similarity to prescription medicines gives herbal medicines the same potential to cause harmful side effects, including negative effects on sexual performance.[21] The large increase in use of herbal medicines, which are widely available over-the-counter and are not under as strict regulatory control as are prescription medicines by governmental agencies such as the FDA, means that their potential adverse effects on sexual performance should be considered. In this book, *Chapter 5* discusses herbs.

Drug-drug & Other Types of Interactions

Even if all of the medicines that a person is taking are appropriate and helpful individually, they can interact in various adverse ways. Such "drug-drug interactions" (DDIs) can occur at any level of drug passage or action in the body: absorption, distribution, metabolism, elimination, or molecular mechanism of action. One of the major processes responsible for adverse DDIs is metabolism. The liver, which is strategically located in the blood circulation so that it can inactivate ingested toxins contains a large quantity of 'drug-metabolizing' enzymes. Most drugs are processed by several of these enzymes and therefore undergo multiple 'biotransformations' and produce multiple metabolites. Metabolic DDIs, particularly those involving the cytochrome P450 system, are the most common, most clinically relevant and most potentially avoidable.[22,23] Some medicines can interfere with the metabolism of others,[24,25] in some cases significantly increasing their concentration in the blood and thereby the adverse effects. The same is true of herbal products and other over-the-counter products.[26-28] Therefore, when we discuss medicine-induced decreased sexual performance in this book, you should take into account everything that you are taking, including herbals and over-the counter-products. And remember, the occurrence of a drug-drug interaction increases with the number of medicines taken. [29]

4

Is Your Med on This List

"Medicine, I have reason since to notice more than once, remains an imperfect art."

– Joan Didion, *Blue Nights*

Pharmaceuticals are the most frequently used therapeutic intervention. Most Americans use some medicines during a typical year at least once and many people use 5 or more on a daily basis. When we say pharmaceuticals, we usually mean drugs, independent of whether they are available over-the-counter or only through a doctor's prescription. For consistency throughout this book, we will use the terms drugs, medicines, or meds instead of pharmaceuticals. It has been estimated that over three-quarters of all doctor visits by patients result in at least one prescription medicine.

Also, we cannot dismiss the importance and potency of over-the-counter (OTC) drugs since many of them began life as prescription drugs, but then after many years of proven safety and effectiveness, they were switched to OTC status. That was the case for most antihistamines for allergies, the drugs for stomach ulcers, and for gastric reflux as well as the creams and ointments for skin inflammation, just to name a few examples.

By the time a person reaches age 50, there is a high probability that

that person is taking a medicine for high blood pressure or diabetes, or for arthritis or for high levels of lipids such as cholesterol. Many others are taking meds for anxiety, depression, low back pain, asthma, gout, GERD (Acid Reflux Disease), COPD (Congestive Obstructive Pulmonary Disease). And it is no longer rare for a patient to have several of these conditions and taking medicines for each of the medical problems.

In this book, we have concentrated on the top approximately 200 best selling medicines in the United States, since those products account for close to 80 percent of all of the OTC drugs sold and medicines dispensed. There are several ways one might use this book to benefit. One avenue is to go directly to Appendix A, and check the the information written on the given pages for their drug of interest. Those page numbers are found after the drug name. The other pathway is for the reader to go directly to the chapter that deals with a given therapeutic area such as depression or heart failure. In that chapter, there will be write-ups for the most commonly used drugs for that medical problem.

A word to the wise is needed here. Your doctor, most likely, prescribed for you the medicines that he or she thought were optimal for you taking into consideration your other conditions, health status, disease severity, family history and the other medicines that you are currently taking. However, if you see a note in the book that your drug interferes with some sexual aspect, your next step is to see whether the other drugs listed in that identical therapeutic area cause the same problems. If there is no mention of sexual problems with one or more of the alternative drugs used for your condition, it seems reasonable that a conversation is in order with your physician to inquire whether one of the other drug products available for your condition might be tried for you. The physician may say that the alternative drugs you mentioned are less potent or are not appropriate for you. However, by mentioning the suspicion you have that your medicines may be interfering with your sexual performance, the physician might check all of the medicines you are using to determine whether another one of your drugs might be the culprit.

Last, the listings in this book are not definitive. At the time the book was completed, we believe that the information presented here was relevant and accurate, but as we all know, new scientific information is announced nearly every day. And we must remember that our sexual performance declines gradually over the years with or without any medicine use. In fact, there may be nothing specific that is wrong. A 75 year-old person does not usually have the stamina, energy, strength, hearing, or visual capabilities of an 18 year old person.

If you find no listing for your drug associated with any sexual performance problem, consider yourself fortunate.

Part Three
Meds Used to Improve Sex

5

Male Performance Enhancers

"Sex at age 90 is like trying to shoot pool with a rope."

– George Burns

Until 1998 we could say with confidence that there were almost no prescription drugs that could improve a man's sex performance and none that could make what was already pretty good into something great. The drug industry had pretty much given up on trying to make any despite the obvious profit enticement. Drug developers tended to believe that the problem of sexual dysfunction was just too complicated a product of mind and body chemistry interaction. Yes there was testosterone (we'll deal with that later) and reports of herbs used in Asia but that was it.

But then, *voila*, it happened again! A drug originally developed to treat one problem began to be reported by physicians to have a side effect that fixed another problem. In clinical trials, it was found that sildenafil, made in England by a Pfizer lab to treat high blood pressure (hypertension) and angina (a heart disease symptom), was having a positive affect on erectile dysfunction. A delighted Pfizer decided to patent it. It was approved by the FDA in the U.S. for erectile dysfunction and branded as Viagra in 1998. Notably, although a prescription only drug, it became very well known as it was advertised on TV by Bob Dole, a former presidential candidate. Soon children were asking their parents, "Daddy, what's priapism?" "Mommy, what's erectile dysfunction."

Of course other pharmaceutical companies wanted some of the action and undertook research to develop competitors. So now in addition to Viagra, we have Cialis, Levitra, and Stendra. In early 2013 Viagra had about 50% of the market, followed by Cialis with about 40%, and Levitra with about 9%. That leaves about 1% for Stendra. These are all in a family of drugs called PDE5 inhibitors. All four of them have similar effects, both positive and adverse, their main differences are in their duration of activity and how fast they work.

This chapter will tell you about the drugs available to treat the primary male sexual problems – erectile dysfunction (ED) and premature ejaculation (PE). These problems are very common. They are associated with age but also with health problems such as diabetes, depression, obesity, prostate cancer surgery, high serum lipid levels. It's estimated that one third of adult males have a health problem affecting their sex performance, sometimes as an adverse effect of the medicine they are taking to treat their health problem.

Men also have age-related lack of lubrication. This problem is treated for both men and women by over-the-counter lubricants and for men lubricated condoms. See *Chapter 16*.

If you're now taking any of the drugs listed above and you simply can't wait to learn about the adverse effects you might have, see the Table at the end of this chapter now. Also, when you get your prescription filled, you should also get a Patient Information Leaflet. Read it!

How Do We Know What Works?
You may want to know how the effectiveness (efficacy) of the male sex performance enhancers is measured. The main areas measured in clinical trials of drugs treating ED are penis erection, erection maintenance (stamina), and satisfaction. There is no lack of measures. A

15-item International Index of Erectile Function (IIEF) includes questions to measure the ability to achieve and maintain an erection and satisfaction. Other measures include Erectile Dysfunction Inventory of Treatment Satisfaction (EDITS), Erection Hardness Score (EHS), Quality of Life Questionnaire (QOL), Sexual Encounter Profile (SEP), Sexual Experience Questionnaire (SEX-Q), global assessment question (GAQ) about erection improvement, quality of erection (QEQ), self-esteem and relationship questionnaire (SEAR), nocturnal penile tumescence (NPT), event logs, general efficacy questions, and partner questionnaires, e.g., the Sexual Life Quality Questionnaire (SLQQ).

Efficacy measures for PE include ejection latency time (ELT) which simply means "How long did it take?," intravaginal ejaculatory latency time (IELT), and a simple scale from "almost never" to "almost always."

Viagra

The generic name for Viagra is sildenafil. Pfizer has managed to hold on to its patent, which was expected to expire in 2012 but now is valid until 2019. Sildenafil is also marketed under the brand name, Revatio, to treat a kind of lung hypertension, and this has provided a rationale for patent extension. As you can imagine, there are many drug companies just panting to put their own generic version of Viagra on the market.

In May of 2013, Pfizer announced that Viagra was available directly from Pfizer including via the Internet. A prescription will still be required. In the first order, the first three of "the little blue pills" will be free with 30% off Pfizer's $25 per pill cost of the next one. Pfizer's justification is that it evaluated 22 Web sites offering Viagra but 80% of them only contained 30-50% of sildenafil, the active ingredient.

Viagra comes in 3 dose sizes, 25, 50, and 100 mg. The 25 mg pill is usually tried first as adverse effects escalate with higher doses.

Of course the big question for men with ED is "How much can Viagra help me?" The many clinical trials reported about 80% of men with ED had improvement compared with men with ED receiving a placebo.[1-4] However, about 25% of the men receiving the placebo also had improvement. As for adverse effects, less than 30% had mild to moderate effects and 10% or less receiving the placebo had them. About 2% taking Viagra dropped out due to a severe adverse effect.

As for men with other health problems, a steady stream of research supports the use of Viagra for ED. For example, a study in 2001 looked at dose differences and included men with diabetes, high blood pressure, a history of pelvic surgery, and heart disease. After 12 weeks 82% had improved erections compared with 24% receiving placebos.[1] In other studies, more than 85% with hypertension had improved ED with Viagra with the usual percent reporting side effects.[5] Men with Type 2 diabetes also may benefit from Viagra.[6] It was also found to help men with early Parkinson's Disease which is often associated with ED, with almost 70% compared with 13% on the placebo reporting Viagra had improved their erections.[7] However, adding testosterone to Viagra was not found to improve ED even in men who had low testosterone.[8]

But ugh!, what about the adverse effects? Of course if you have any of the four serious ones (Table 5.1 at end of chapter), they are immediate game changers. You must call your doctor at once. Not in Table 5.1, but recently published, a study reported an association of Viagra use with an increased risk of melanoma, which is a serious skin cancer. The authors state: "Although this study is insufficient to alter clinical recommendations, we support a need for continued investigation of this association".[9] The same risk might apply to similar-acting drugs, but it has not been studied. If you have any of the other less serious side effects, affecting about 2% of users and often diminishing with time, to about 20% who have a headache, you decide. Is your headache worth the ED fix? Is the classic female excuse, "Not tonight dear I have a headache" now coming from the other side of the bed?

But on to the second male performance enhancer appearing on the market.

Levitra

Levitra (vardenafil) was approved by the FDA in 2003 and its patent expires in 2018. Dose strengths are 2.5, 5, 10, and 20 mg.

If you can't wait an hour, Levitra may be for you. Levitra comes in two dose forms, one is enteric coated and one dissolves in the mouth.[9] The 10 mg one, dissolving in the mouth, called the orodispersable form, was successful in one study within 15 minutes for more than 60% of men with ED.[11] Success with the coated version was pretty fast too. Within 30 minutes, either form succeeded in more than 70% of men taking it whether 10 or 20 mg. Another study found it successful for men of any age and regardless of their ED severity.[12]

One study reported that when men took Levitra, it improved their sexual function and their female partners reported it improved their sex life quality as well.[13]

What about adverse effects? Adverse effects were found to be the same with either the orally dissolving or the coated form.[14] Not only does Levitra work fast, its adverse effects are mild-moderate and usually decrease after continued use.[15] The most common are headache, flushing, stuffy or runny nose, and upset stomach. About a fifth of users have one or more of these. Also, in addition to reported faster onset than Viagra, Levitra has less risk of vision-related adverse effects.[16]

A review of studies in 2009 stated that men with the other health problems often associated with ED - diabetes, hypertension, high blood lipids - and who take other medicines for these problems, might favor Levitra as their first choice.[17] It works and has a favorable safety profile. However, in men with diabetes which had led to ED, Cialis and Levitra were found equally effective.[18] Both drugs were well tolerated with no serious side effects.

Almost 40% of men with high blood pressure who took Levitra every day for five weeks achieved success after failing to respond when using it on-demand.[19]

And for healthy obese men with PE, Levitra increased sexual performance and increased self-esteem.[20] In another study of men with PE, Levitra and Zoloft (an antidepressant) were compared.[21] Levitra increased intravaginal ejaculation time from just under a minute to 5.1 minutes and Zoloft increased it to 3.1 minutes on average. Another study measured ejaculation time achieved by masturbation, and reported that Levitra increased the average time from 1.3 to 3.2 minutes.[22]

For men with shrinking gonads, a combination of Levitra and testosterone was found more effective than either of these alone.[23]

Cialis

Cialis (tadalafil) was approved by the FDA for erectile dysfunction in 2008. Its patent expires in 2020 so don't expect a cheaper generic before then. The advantage of Cialis is that it's a once-daily dose eliminating the need to plan ahead.[24] You may have seen some of the commercials promoting Cialis, one featuring a couple hanging laundry to dry who just can't wait an hour. Also, its lower dose compared with Viagra may result in fewer adverse effects.

Cialis is available in 5, 10, and 20 mg tablets. Does it work? The FDA reported that 22 clinical trials involving more than 4,000 men for up to 24 weeks found it effective for ED. About 3% of men dropped out of the trials due to adverse effects but about 2% on the placebo also dropped out citing adverse effects. A daily dose of 5 mg was found to significantly improve self-esteem, confidence, sexual relationship satisfaction, and nocturnal penile tumescence.[25] Another study found it to work and to be well-tolerated with low rates of common adverse effects such as flushing and headache and no significant differences between the 5 mg and 20 mg dose.[26] Also, no differences were found between improvement of ED, adverse effects, and satisfaction with daily dosing of Cialis versus using it on-demand as is done with Viagra.[27]

As for men with other health problems, Cialis plus testosterone was better than testosterone alone for treating shrinking sex organs in old and middle-aged men.[28] Taking 20 mg of Cialis daily was more successful in treating ED in men with high serum lipids than taking a statin drug such as Lipitor alone.[29] In a study of more than 100 men who had prostate surgery and developed ED, 87% improved compared with 25% who improved in the placebo group.[30] Also, long-term treatment with Cialis improved ED in men with pulmonary arterial hypertension for a year.[31]

A review of studies in the medical literature since 2000 concluded that Levitra was preferred over Viagra and Cialis.[32] Why? Mainly because of the longer duration of action that increased couple's freedom in sexual life.

Stendra

Stendra (avanafil) is the newest arrow in the ED drug quiver. It was approved in the spring of 2012 and comes in dose sizes of 50, 100, and 200 mg. Compared to the other ED treatment drugs on the market, it rates high in effectiveness and safety.[33,34] A study compared Stendra with Viagra.[34] It showed that peak response occurred at 20-40 minutes after dosing while with Viagra, peak response was from 60-120 minutes. In another study including men with diabetes, successful intercourse occurred as early as 15 minutes with Stendra and could still occur as late as 6 hours or more after dosing.[35] In addition, its adverse effects tend to be mild and similar to those associated with the three other ED treatment drugs. In one study, face flushing was the most common, occurring in 7-15% of men, and no one had a vision problem.[35]

The "take home message" seems to be that Stendra, which displays faster onset of action, and favorable adverse-effects compared with the other available ED drugs, offers an alternative first line treatment option for men with ED.[36]

Premature Ejaculation (PE)

In addition to Levitra and possibly the other Viagra-like drugs, another choice to increase ejaculation time is condoms. Not just any condom, but ones lined with a numbing substance, most often benzocaine. This is a trade-off. Yes, more inside time but also less feeling.

Treating Nerve Damage ED

As for men with spinal cord injuries who often have decreased sexual function, a review of studies indicates that Viagra, Cialis, and Levitra are not different in effectiveness or satisfaction[37] and we would not expect it with Stendra either. These drugs are first line ED therapy for these men but encouraging results are also reported for men with Parkinson's and Multiple Sclerosis.[38] They are limited for men with other central nerve damage for various reasons, such as depression, being the cause of their ED and low desire.

Testosterone

Suffering from "Low T"? If yes, you may have small gonads caused by lack of testicles producing enough sex hormones. A review of studies from 1969-2010 on testosterone replacement therapy (TRT) concluded that low T is very common in aging men and is associated with physical and sexual weakness.[39] TRT reduces body fat, increases leanness, bone density, and symptoms of depression. TRT alone, or in combination with one of the drugs as discussed above, is first-line treatment for men with ED. However, beware. The number of T prescriptions has tripled since 2001 and a recent study reported that taking it more than quadrupled the number of adverse cardiovascular events in men over 65. Also, taking it may reduce the normal production of testosterone in the body. It is recommended that physicians test the T levels in their patients before prescribing it, but alas, many physicians do not do so, resulting in overdoses.[40]

Testosterone now comes as a patch, injection, implant, gel, or solution applied to the skin. It is usually applied once a day on any part of the body. Brand names of the gel are Androderm, Androgel, Fortesta, and Testim, but it is also available generically as testosterone. The brand name of the transdermal solution is Axiron and of the implanted pellet, Testopel. Names of the oral tablets are Android 10, Android 20, Methyltestosterone, and Testred. Names of the injectable version are Delastryl, Depotestosterone, Testosterone Cypionate, and Testosterone Enanthate. And yes, you need a prescription to get it.

Users are cautioned to make sure it doesn't get on females and children.

Supplements

A supplement form of L-arginine may help men with ED. L-arginine is an amino acid in plant and animal products, meat, poultry, fish, and nuts. In a study of 50 men with ED who took either 5 grams of L-arginine per day or placebo for 6 weeks, more men taking L-arginine improved compared to those taking the placebo.[41] However, although L-arginine may be safe in the short term, it can cause a number of side effects, such as indigestion, nausea, headache, bloating, diarrhea, and gout.

Herbs

You may have taken a cruise and when you got off the ship in a foreign port at the end of the pier you found stands and/or shops offering "natural Viagra." Cheap too. But do they work? The answer is "maybe, but not very likely." Studies in China, India, Iran, South Africa, and South Korea have shown that a few herbs can help male infertility and ED. Most of them touted for these problems either do not help or have not been studied. Purchasers can't tell if these "over-the-counter" herbs have any active ingredient or even if they are what they are labeled to be. Is that really maca or ginseng or saffron or whatever?

A review done in the UK involving studies of older patients, using complementary and alternative medicine (CAM) for sexual dysfunction, concluded most of the studies were biased and only a very few showed any positive results.[42] The FDA considers herbs to be naturally occurring plants and does not approve them any more than it does parsley or thyme or any other herbs you buy in a grocery store. If you live in, for example China, and have a trusted health care provider, then maybe you might use an herb. But otherwise, buyer beware. You have no way of knowing what you are buying or if what you are buying is contaminated.

Counterfeits

A justification for Pfizer selling Viagra directly was that about 80% of Viagra sold on 22 Web sites was fake and only contained 30-50% of the active drug.

Counterfeit drugs are a dangerous growing problem.[43] Millions of counterfeit male performance enhancers, Viagra and its cousins, are seized each year and account for most counterfeit seizures. Analysis of these seized drugs showed active ingredients varying from 0% to over 200% of the labeled dose and many with harmful contaminants. Contaminants included talcum powder, paint, printer ink, and other active ingredients you don't want.

The Future

2018 is the earliest any of the drugs described above goes off patent and will be available generically, which usually means cheaper. Currently there are many ongoing clinical trials of drugs to help men with sexual dysfunction. Most are in the same drug family as those discussed above. The goal is to produce ones that act quickly, always work, last a long time, have few if any adverse-effects, and seem worth the money. Eventually, look to see these available over-the-counter.

Table 5.1. Adverse effects of male performance enhancers.*

Serious Effects – Call doctor at once	Viagra	Cialis	Levitra	Stendra
Erection painful or lasts more than 4 hours	X	X	X	X
Decrease or loss of vision	X	X	X	X
Decrease or loss of hearing	X	X	X	X
Ringing in ears	X			
Effects which may go away. If do not or severe, tell doctor				
Headache	X	X	X	X
Upset stomach	X	X	X	
Diarrhea	X			
Flushing	X	X	X	X
Dizzyness	X		X	X
Pain in stomach, back, muscles, arms, legs		X		X
Stuffy or runny nose		X	X	X
Upper respiratory tract infection				X
Flu-like symptoms			X	X
Rash	X			
Vision: blurred, sensitive to light, or change in color	X			

* These adverse effects are reported by the US Food and Drug Administration. They are more likely to occur with higher doses. Those which may go away were reported in more than 2% of users in clinical trials.

6

Female Performance Enhancers

*"Love looks not with the eyes, but with the mind,
And therefore is winged Cupid painted blind."*

– William Shakespeare, *A Midsummer Night's Dream*

As you might have guessed there are many more articles about males than there are about females in the sexual dysfunction professional literature. One reason is that men often suffer from lack of performance but seldom from lack of desire. Women may suffer from either or both. Apparently it's been easier for scientists to develop drugs to treat male performance problems than to develop ones for female performance problems. And although some women need treatment for lack of desire, developing a treatment for it has proved difficult. Scientists know that desire and performance are connected and affected by dopamine and serotonin, which are neurotransmitters in the brain, but the connections have not proven easy to understand. Without understanding, a problem is hard to fix.

Lack of desire is believed to be the most common form of female sex dysfunction – affecting up to 10% of US women.[1] Its defined medically as "persistent or recurrent deficiency or absence of sexual fantasies and thoughts, and/or desire for, or receptivity to, sexual activity, which causes personal distress or interpersonal difficulties and is not caused by a medical condition or drug." However, the percentage may be much higher as doctors often don't ask and their female patients are often reluctant to volunteer sex related information.

The other major areas in female sexual dysfunction are lack of orgasm and age-related pain during sex, which the medical community calls dyspareunia.

Although none are available now, new drugs are undergoing clinical trials that may help women with both lack of desire and lack of performance. For age-related sex problems, there are many prescription estrogens (female hormones), some containing other drugs as well. See estrogen list at the end of this chapter. There are also many over-the-counter lubricants available. Since they are used by both men and women, lubricants are dealt with in *Chapter 16*.

This chapter will tell you about estrogens and what's in the research pipeline. It will also tell you about how age, medications, and other health issues impact female sex problems.

How Do We Know What Works?

As two areas in female's sexual disorder are treated, two kinds of measures are used to determine if a drug works. To measure lack of desire, HSDD (hypoactive sexual-desire disorder) is commonly used. A newer measure is SIAD (sexual interest/arousal disorder). There are also questionnaires and interviews. For example, interviews are used to help explain answers obtained by the FSFI (Female Sexual Function Index) questionnaire. Other questionnaires are the FSAD (Female Sexual Arousal Disorder), which measures changes in sexual behavior, and the SSE, which asks about sexual satisfaction events. Also there is the DISF (DeRogatis Inventory of Sexual Function), which has been used when sexual disorder is caused by depression. The DSDS (Decreased Sexual Desire Screener) was developed for health care providers who are not trained in FSD (Female Sexual Dysfunction). When measuring Viagra like or other drugs for increasing blood flow, the genital area may be monitored with machines. There's one to measure blood volume in the clitoris, one to measure blood volume in the vagina, and another to measure skin conductance.[2]

What's the Cause?
Causes of low desire include other medical problems, medications, surgeries, psychosocial factors, and increased age.

A contributing factor to females' sexual dysfunction can be erectile dysfunction (ED) in their partners. One study gave the FSFI questionnaire to women whose spouses were taking a Viagra-like performance enhancer.[3] Before the men started taking the drug, 50% of the women scored in the dysfunctional range. But, after the men took the drug for six months, almost 60% of these women scored in the functional range.

Medicines taken for mental disorders such as depression and schizophrenia may affect lubrication, orgasm, sexual arousal, and overall sexual satisfaction. Switching to a different medicine may help.[4,5] Millions of women are treating depression with antidepressants and these affect serotonin in the brain which is involved in desire.

Prescription Drugs
After the Viagra-type drugs hit the market, physicians began to say, "Where are the drugs to help our female patients?" So the drugs known to help men's sexual dysfunction were given to women to see if they would help women too. These were primarily testosterone and Viagra-like drugs.

<u>Testosterone.</u> Doctors figured that if the primary male hormone, testosterone, helped men, why not try it on women too? Women do have testosterone, but much less than men. You just don't want to give women so much more that they develop a deep voice, whiskers, and male-pattern baldness.

Oral contraceptives were known to depress testosterone so levels were studied before and three months after women began taking them.[6] The oral contraceptives depressed testosterone in the women taking them, however, the reduced testosterone did not affect their enjoyment of sexual activity with a partner. Some women did and some didn't have fewer sexual thoughts. Overall, the results were consistent with the idea that some women are more sensitive to testosterone levels than are others.

Doctors awaited results from clinical trials on LibiGel.[7] LibiGel, which contained testosterone, reached women's blood stream through their skin. It was supposed to treat female's lack of interest by increasing the dopamine rush in their brains. Alas, it was not approved by the FDA because in its clinical trials, it didn't work better than a placebo.

<u>Viagra-like.</u> And for females, why not a Viagra-like drug? Seems logical. But remember that the Viagra-like drugs do not produce erections in men unless their brains send a message, "Yes, I want to have sex." In men, this "yes" is apparently in their brains more often and louder than it is in female brains. So far, for women with sexual disorders, it remains uncertain whether a Viagra-like drug works better than a placebo.

In one study, women with desire and/or arousal disorder got testosterone and on a different day, testosterone and Viagra. On another day they got placebos. It was known that many women with sexual dysfunction have low response to sexual stimulation. Two measures of this were used, a measure of sensitivity to sexual content and the other measured genital and subjective response to erotic film clips. The women with low sensitivity to sexual content at the outset increased it after receiving testosterone, but testosterone decreased the sensitivity in the women who had high sensitivity at the outset. When both testosterone and Viagra were taken, they improved genital response and the subjective measure in the low sensitivity group, but had no effect in the group with high sensitivity at the outset. The take-away is that this combination may only help women who don't respond well to sexual cues.[8]

In another study of men and women with sex problems related to depression, Viagra and Levitra helped the men but not the women. Only an antidepressant helped the women.[9]

A review of the scientific literature concluded that Viagra, while well-tolerated, offers little or no benefit in most women with sexual disorder.[10]

Coming Down the Pipeline

Two drugs, Librido and Libridos, are in clinical trials. Although these are often referred to as "the female Viagra" this is wrong. Viagra works on arteries and causes blood to flow to the penis. Librido and Libridos have ingredients that are supposed to affect the brain and stimulate desire. They are intended to be lust pills, especially for women 20-60 years old who have lost interest.

Even when Viagra-like drugs have increased blood flow to female genitals, it hasn't turned on the "yes" in female brains. So why not? Dopamine, a neurotransmitter, radiates desire, the "yes, I want to have sex," message in the brain. The hormone, testosterone, and another neurotransmitter, serotonin, also are players. Testosterone stimulates dopamine and serotonin moderates self-control. These need to be balanced. Too much serotonin and the result is lack of lust. A goal of Librido and Libridos is to affect this balance and generate "turn-ons" in female brains.

Librido and Libridos have two active chemicals that work together to affect the balance between dopamine and serotonin in the brain so that dopamine overcomes the "let's not say yes" effect of serotonin. Both Librido and Libridos have testosterone in a mint flavored coating which melts in the mouth. Inside the coating, the timed-release Librido tablet is Viagra-like and intended to send blood to female genitals. Awareness in the brain is supposed to stimulate its dopamine rush. In Libridos, the inner timed release tablet contains buspirone instead of the Viagra-like compound. Buspirone's short-term action suppresses serotonin in the brain so that dopamine can have more effect.

Preliminary clinical trials for these two drugs are reported to be positive in the areas of desire and increased orgasm. However, for the FDA to approve them, the results of a larger study must be positive and also show that these drugs are safe. Don't look for them to be on the market before 2016.

Another drug undergoing clinical trials is filbanserin. In three studies it was given to women with low sexual desire disorder.[11-13] It was reported to be well-tolerated and to show significant improvements in satisfying sexual events and sexual-desire, and reductions in distress related to low sexual-desire. The female sex hormones, estrogen and progesterone, are produced by the ovaries. These hormones regulate menstruation and are responsible for secondary female characteristics. Their role in sexual desire and functioning is unclear, but they do maintain the lining of the vagina. During menopause, less estrogen is produced, and the vaginal lining becomes thin and dry (senile vaginitis) so that sexual intercourse is painful and unpleasant (dyspareunia).

What a dirty trick nature played on women. Just when they no longer have to worry about getting pregnant without a condom, the areas dry up that help them enjoy sex. To treat this and to treat hot flashes, women are often given estrogens to replace those that are no longer being produced by the body. For age-related lack of lubricaton, see the list at the end of this chapter. They are all only available by prescription.

In fact men also have age-related loss of lubrication. Their only fall back is over-the-counter lubricants that are dealt with for men and women in *Chapter 16*.

Estrogens

At one time well over half of menopausal women took estrogens, primarily to control hot flashes, and one of them, Premarin, was one of the top twenty drugs sold in the United States. Prescriptions fell off when a national study tracking women's health reported that estrogens taken by mouth were associated with an increased risk of stroke, breast cancer, and cardiovascular events.

For age related lack of lubrication and painful intercourse, estrogens are usually applied in a vaginal cream but sometimes a vaginal ring is used. Premarin Vaginal Cream is the most common. It contains conjugated estrogens and other ingredients. Conjugated estrogens are a mix of naturally occurring forms of estrogens obtained from the urine of pregnant mares. The primary estrogens present are sodium estrone sulfate and sodium equilin sulfate.

Many brands of esterified estrogens are also prescribed to help reduce symptoms of menopause such as hot flashes and vaginal dryness. Many of them also contain methyltestosterone. They are usually taken by mouth. Esterification is a process that changes estrogens to improve how they are orally absorbed and extends their half-life in the body so they don't have to be taken as often. If injected, esterification results in the estrogens being absorbed more slowly in the body, which extends their half-life.

An oral tablet, Osphena (ospemifene), taken once a day, was approved by the FDA in early 2013 to reduce pain (dyspareunia) associated with vulval and vaginal atrophy. It is an estrogen receptor modulator which acts like estrogen to thicken the wall of the vagina. However the FDA's black-box warning states that it could lead to blood clots and endometrial cancer. Other risks, primarily cardiovascular such as stroke, occur less often than those associated with estrogen-therapy alone. Nevertheless, this drug should be used for the shortest amount of time due to associated adverse effects.[14]

If you wish to treat symptoms occurring only in and around the vagina, products applied directly inside the vagina such as Premarin Vaginal Cream should be considered before those taken by mouth, absorbed through the skin, injected, or after taking Osphena for a short time.

Some orally taken estrogens are in combination with other drugs such as meprobamate which treats anxiety. Various estrogen medications in addition to conjugated estrogens are treatment options. They include estradiol and estriol tablets and vaginal creams, a sustained release-estradiol vaginal ring, and combinations with methytestosterone which may prove safe and efficacious to treat age-related vaginal atrophy, but more clinical studies are needed.[14]

Serious adverse effects have been related to estrogens. Symptoms that should alert users to call their doctor include: breast lumps, vaginal bleeding, dizziness and fainting, severe headaches, shortness of breath, leg pains, vision or voice changes, vomiting, yellowing of skin, eyes, or nail beds. Side effects that are less serious and may go away are: headache, breast pain, stomach cramps/bloating, nausea, hair loss, fluid retention, and vaginal yeast infection.

Summary

For age-related sexual disorder, there are estrogens and lubricants. For lack of orgasm and/or sexual desire, drugs are in the pipeline.

Estrogens	
Brand Names	**Active Ingredients**
Amnestrogen	esterified estrogens
Cenestin	conjugated synthetic A estrogens
Covaryx	esterified estrogens, methyltestosterone
Essian	esterified estrogens, methyltestosterone
Estratest	esterified estrogens, methyltestosterone

Estrogens	
Femtest	esterified estrogens, methytestosterone
Enjuvia	conjugated synthetic B estrogens
Estrace tablets	estradiol
Estratab	esterified estrogens
Evex	esterified estrogens
Femogen	esterified estrogens
Menest	esterified estrogens
Menogen	esterified estrogens, methyltestosterone
Premarin cream	conjugated estrogens
Premarin with Methyltestosterone	conjugated estrogens
Syntest	esterified estrogens, methyltestosterone

7

Aphrodiasics and Placebos

"Don't you remember that love, like medicine, is only the art of encouraging nature?"

— Pierre Choderlos de Laclos, *Les Liaisons Dangereuses*

We have all seen advertisements promoting products that will help you delay your climax in order to coincide with that of your partner, make even the limpest of men powerful, enable one to go on and on and on, cause the penis to get harder and larger for a prolonged period of time, and awaken and produce sexual desires in men and women alike. While the advertisements varied about the products and their promises, they all shared two characteristics. The advertised products were expensive and somewhere in the printed ad, it said "Placebo."

One must assume that many people responded to these ads, otherwise the products' manufacturers would not have been able to afford to continue the expensive advertising campaigns. Several explanations come to mind. The first market may be for practical jokers who bought these products as birthday gag gifts for their aging golf buddies, or as silly presents for bridegrooms. But surely some people bought these products for themselves without knowing the meaning of the word "placebo." And surely some understood the meaning of the word, and also knew about the Federal Trade Commission (FTC) regulations about truthfulness in advertising, but who found that the products did what they claimed. How can that last situation be true? The answer lies in the power of expectations, beliefs, and attitudes to shape reality. That is the placebo effect.

The word placebo comes from the Latin verb meaning "to please." A placebo is nothing more than a fake medicine, usually a tablet or capsule that contains either harmless, inert ingredients such as sugar or flour, or an injection containing only salt water.[1] Also, some placebo products have impressive lists of vitamins, minerals, and other compounds all in subclinical doses where there can't be any realistic expectation of any pharmacologic action.

Strange as it might seem, fake medicines and fake sex aids can work. A declining sexual ardor can be revived by the belief that the pill is a potent aphrodisiac. Indeed, placebos probably "work" better for sex problems than in any other area of human concern, because of the predominant part the mind plays in sexual desire and performance. Placebos, when prescribed or administered by physicians can be very powerful "medicines." An appreciation of the power of placebos and the placebo effect can help one understand not only why people have believed in aphrodisiacs for so many years, and indeed, why they "work," but why the response to drugs that are supposed to affect a person's sexual desire and performance is so varied and unpredictable. An understanding of the placebo effect may also convince you why it is not possible to evaluate a drug's pharmacological effect on sexual function without a properly designed "double-blind" study.

Doctors do not give sugar pills or salt solutions for sex problems or any other type of problem very often. They don't use placebos because they know what the patient's reaction will be when the patient learns about the deceit by the doctor. Moreover, doctors are not able to accurately predict how well a placebo will work for any given patient. Plus in our advanced society, a doctor is expected to determine what the medical problem is, and to prescribe a drug that is specifically formulated to treat that exact problem. It is easy to see how a doctor charging a fee to a patient, and using fake drugs or a placebo, could be viewed as a quack. The placebo effect is described as any effect attributed to a pill, potion, or procedure, but not to its pharmacodynamic or specific properties. What this means is that the color, shape, taste of the medicine, or the environment, including the personality of the doctor, can have a powerful effect on patients' perceptions of the success of their therapy.[2]

The placebo effect has been described as an example of the mind fooling the body. Examples abound. Placebos have been reported in the scientific literature to cure fever, headache, coughs, colds, insomnia, angina pain, postoperative pain, and even warts. It is important that the doctor, as well as the patient, have faith in the therapy to mobilize the placebo effect. Doctors and other healthcare providers employ the therapeutic assistance of the placebo effect by showing an interest in the patient's welfare, and trying to reduce the patient's anxiety by asking about work or the family or a pet.

So, what do we know about aphrodisiacs or the placebo effect? The answer is a lot and a little. We do know that when people have a high level of confidence in a therapy, they often believe that it is effective, even if scientific knowledge and experience contradict that confidence. People want to believe in something even when conventional medicine tells them the words that no one wants to hear, "I'm sorry but there is nothing further that can be done." That is why patients visit various types of unconventional healers in Mexico or elsewhere, in the hope that some therapy unknown to local physicians and surgeons, but known to their friends or neighbors, might be beneficial.[3]

In recent years, the pharmaceutical industry has developed clinically proven therapies for erectile dysfunction, for low testosterone levels, and for a few other related products, but that has not diminished the number of advertisements we still are exposed to, promoting greater sexual performance for men and women.

Our advice is to seriously doubt the claims made by advertisers for sexual performance enhancing products when those products contain mostly vitamins and minerals, or herbal products. However, if you know someone who claims great personal benefit in the sexual domain from banana peel extract and peanut shell juice, the best thing you can do for that friend is not to interfere and let him go along with his beliefs, since it is not likely hurting anyone. But please urge him to abstain from products made from horns, penises, and testicles, because they do harm the animals they have been taken from.

Part Four
Contraception

8

The Pill and Other Female Contraceptives: Can They Affect Your Sex Life?

"Political analysts say the key voting bloc could be birth control moms. Birth control moms are women who use birth control, but apparently not correctly."

— Conan O'Brien

Oral Contraceptives

COMBINATION PILLS

Alesse, Apri, Aviane, Brevicon, Demulen, Desogen, Estrostep, Estrostep Fe, Genora, Jenest-28, Levlen, Levora, Lo/Ovra, Loestrin, Loestrin Fe, Loestrin 24 Fe, Low-Ogestrel, Microgestin, Microgestin Fe, Mircette, Modicon, Necon 10/11, Nordette, Norinyl, Nortrel, Ogestrel, Ortho Tri-Cyclen, Ortho-Cept, Ortho-Cyclen, Ortho-Novum, Ortho-Novum 10/11, Ortho-Novum 7/7/7, Ovcon, Ovral, Tri-Levlen, Tri-Norinyl, Triphasil, Trivora, Yasmin, Yaz, Zovia

EXTENDED CYCLE PILLS

Lybrel, Seasonale, Seasonique

MINI PILLS
Micronor, Nor-QD, Ovrette

What's the difference? Mini Pills contain only a single hormone ingredient, a form of progestin, while the combination pills contain both the progestin and estrogen hormones. Traditionally, 21 of the 28 pills in the combination packs contain the hormones and 7 are placebos, so that they simulate a normal 28-day menstrual cycle. Extended-cycle packs have pills for three months, and for two of the months, all 28 pills contain hormones. As a result, menstruation should only occur in one of every three months.

Most oral contraceptives contain a progestin and an estrogen. Estrogen occurs naturally in the body, but progestins are synthetic variations of the naturally occurring progesterone. Progesterone is not absorbed when it is taken orally, so synthetic forms, such as levonorgestrel that can be absorbed, are put in the pill instead.

Why take a Mini – also known as POPs (progestin only pills)? Because they can be used by women who shouldn't take the combination contraceptives, such as those who have migraine headaches, high blood pressure, or a history of blood clots, and cigarette smokers over 35. Also, women who are breast-feeding can use POPs, since they will not harm the baby and may actually help increase the amount of milk. POPs have other benefits. They decrease menstrual blood flow and cramps, and they reduce the risk of anemia, endometrial cancer, and pelvic inflammatory infection. Ovulation returns quickly after discontinuing POPs and they do not affect fertility.

How Does the Pill Work?
The oral contraceptive pill works by tricking the pituitary gland into believing that the body is pregnant. Yep. When the gland accepts this, it refuses to send out the two hormones, FSH and LH, that signal the ovary to release one of its eggs (an ovum). If there are no eggs released, there can be no pregnancy. *Voila.*

Briefly, this is how the normal menstrual cycle works:

1. The pituitary gland sends out FSH & LH.

2. FSH & LH tell the ovaries to release an ovum and to produce estrogen.

3. The ovum is released and the ovaries begin to produce progesterone and estrogen.

4. Progesterone and estrogen tell the pituitary gland to stop releasing FSH & LH.

5. If the ovum is not fertilized, the ovaries decrease their production of estrogen and progesterone, and menstruation occurs.

6. The low level of estrogen and progesterone tells the pituitary to start sending out FSH & LH, and start the cycle over again.

If estrogen is given at the start of the cycle, no ovum matures sufficiently to be released, because the estrogen tells the pituitary gland not to send out the FSH and LH that are responsible for the maturation and release of the ovum. The progestin component of the pill, along with the estrogen, prepares the lining of the uterus for the baby just in case there is one. After three weeks of taking the pill, the woman stops taking it. The decrease of estrogen and progestin signals the uterus that there's no baby after all, and the lining of the uterus is sloughed off in the process known as menstruation.

Can Hormone Contraceptives Affect My Sex Life?

Since their introduction in the 1960s, oral contraceptives have been taken by millions of women. Very soon after their introduction there were reports stating that 'the pill' decreases women's sexual desire.[1] At first, there were just a few letters to medical journals saying that the pill depressed some patients and also decreased their libido. Other doctors countered by saying that, in their patients, the pill had the opposite effect. It was in effect an aphrodisiac. Others said that with so many millions of women taking the pill, of course there would be some women who would find it a depressant, and who was to say that the decrease in libido reported by some women was related to the pill? Maybe some women had deep feelings of guilt about using any contraceptive, and the guilt did it. Or, maybe guilt and fear about the new freedom the pill gave women was to blame. Or perhaps suppressed anger about having lost the excuse not to have sex, which they really didn't like anyway.[2] Times have changed. As an example, the official FDA approved label ('package insert') for Loestrin states: "Patients becoming significantly depressed while taking oral contraceptives should stop the medication and use an alternate method of contraception in an attempt to determine whether the symptom is drug related." As for the claim that the pill had aphrodisiac effects, the counter argument was that those who seemed to have an increase in libido after taking the pill weren't really sexually stimulated, they were just so relieved at not risking pregnancy, that they were much less sexually inhibited. [3]

Although medical journal reports of the pill's depressing libido were few relative to the number of women on the pill, they may have represented the experience of many more, simply because few pill-prescribing doctors asked their patients about their sexual feelings or problems, and few women brought the subject up themselves. Sound familiar?

As the number of reports in medical journals increased, underground reports of the pill's effects began to accumulate and spread. Some of the shared experience moved into the public arena as women formed 'consciousness-raising' groups in the sixties and early seventies. Women began to demand a greater input into decisions that affected their bodies. They also wanted to know about the risks associated with the various methods of contraception so that they could make up their own minds. More information on 'the pill' began to appear in women's magazines and books about women's health, not all written by doctors, but by the users.

One would think that a question about a side effect of a drug taken by millions of women would stimulate dozens of research projects. But no. Even by the late seventies, only a few large, well-designed scientific inquiries had been made into the effect of the pill on women's sexual functioning. Of course such studies are difficult to do because it's unethical to have a double-blind study with half of the women taking placebos. Because of the prominent place that psychological factors play in sexual activity, it isn't valid simply to have women take the pill, then ask them about changes in their sexual feelings or activity, and infer from their answers that the pill caused those feelings or activity. The scientific way is to have a double-blind clinical trial and to randomize women into a pill group and a placebo group. Then ask each group about their feelings and sex activity, and compare them. This method looks good on paper, but what woman would want to volunteer for an experiment in which she had even a one in ten chance of getting a sugar pill instead of a contraceptive pill? Another research method is to compare the feelings and activity of women taking birth control pills with those of women using other methods of contraception, such as an intrauterine device (IUD) or the diaphragm. And yet another research method is to have both the pill- and placebo-taking groups use other non-hormonal contraceptive methods at the same time as taking actual pills or placebo, for example, condoms.

Eventually it became known that women who take the pill increase their chance of a stroke, a pulmonary embolism, or a heart attack, any of which can be fatal, and that smoking increases these risks. Printed warnings about these risks must now be given out with oral contraceptives by pharmacists.

A change in sex drive is sometimes mentioned as an occasional reaction to the pill that has not been proven to be directly associated with the pill. But there are scientific reasons for believing that the pill may depress sexual function. For example, one of the common components of the pill, ethinyl estradiol, is used to decrease hypersexuality in men. Another drug, cyproterone acetate, is a close chemical cousin of progestin, which is in all of the oral contraceptives. Cyproterone acetate has been used to treat male hypersexuality, sexual delinquency, and premature sexual development. It reduces the number of sexual thoughts and sexual activity in men and boys. If the progestin depresses sexual function in men, there is reason to believe that it might do it in women too.

Will Hormone Contraceptives Affect My Sex Life?

You probably can't predict whether the pill will affect you sexually. Depending on which medical journal article you read, depression occurs in from about 5% to almost 50% of women who take the pill. Depression almost always affects people, both men and women, sexually. Doctors don't like to warn women that the pill can depress them and their sexual feelings, because they know that a suggestion by an authority figure like a doctor is very powerful, and if a doctor tells a woman that a medicine is going to depress her sexual desire or ability to achieve orgasms, she'll expect it and it becomes much more likely to happen.

Although only a few large well-controlled studies have been conducted since the female hormone contraceptives came on the market, the studies that examined the effect of them on women's sexual desire and function have been published in peer-reviewed professional journals. The authors of a review of 30 studies reported their conclusions about the relationship between the pill and sexual desire (libido).[4] In the 17 studies that asked women after they took the pill about its past effect, most reported an increase in libido. In contrast, in the 4 studies that asked women taking the pill to report in the future about effects, most reported that there was little change. The results from the 5 studies that randomized women into pill- and placebo-groups were mixed. In the most recent of these studies, a decrease in libido among the pill users compared with the placebo users was reported. The authors of the review paper stated: "Over-all, women experience positive effects, negative effects, as well as no effect on libido during OC [oral contraceptive] use". Another review looked at

7 small studies that tried to determine if adverse effects were related to the hormonal action of the pills or were a psychological response to behavior when on the pill.[5] The authors concluded that there was no relationship between hormone levels and emotional feelings. Women given a placebo reported similar adverse effects as those taking an actual pill. An additional review of 36 studies involving 8,422 women taking combined progestin and estrogen oral contraceptive pills found 85% of the women reported no increase or no change in sexual desire despite having a decrease in plasma levels of free testosterone.[6] One review simply concluded: "There appears to be mixed effects on libido, with a small percentage of women experiencing an increase or a decrease, and the majority being unaffected".[7]

Since there are many oral contraceptives, with various combinations, forms and doses of progestin and estrogen in them, women having problems with sexual desire or function are urged to tell their prescribing healthcare provider and ask for a change. Consider the study of 22 healthy women taking the contraceptive pill Yasmin which concluded that this pill: "...is associated with increased pain during intercourse, with decreased libido and spontaneous arousability, and with diminished frequency of sexual intercourse and orgasm".[8] Surely women affected this way should try something else.

Besides the possible loss of libido, both estrogen and progestin have side effects that are not considered serious by many doctors, but may be unpleasant for the women who take them. The estrogen component may cause nausea, vomiting, and breast tenderness. The progestin component may cause headache, dizziness, depression, apathy, and fatigue. Weight gain and retention of fluids are also common. These effects may subside after the user's body gets used to (tolerates) the pill.

What Should I Do?
The decision to take or not to take the pill, or other contraceptive delivering the hormones in the pill, is one of the most serious decisions

a woman makes. The plus side is, if taken according to directions, the chance of a pregnancy is virtually zero.

Remember, too, that some women actually find that these pills increase their sexual desire. This is almost certainly partly related to the effect of being freed of the fear of pregnancy. Without such a fear, women can feel uninhibited, and their natural feelings can be fully expressed.

If you are a young woman twenty-five or less, taking the pill is an easier choice than if you are older. Women who are over forty should consult their doctor. They most certainly should not do so if they smoke. Not only are general and sexual depression more likely, but the risk of stroke, heart attack, and side effects are markedly increased. No woman of any age should take the pill if she has any of the following: a history of thromboembolic disease (blood clots in the veins), liver disease, cancer, tumors in the uterus, migraine headache, asthma, epilepsy, or any kind of blood disease.

How about the use of the pill plus a condom? Women who used either or both were asked about their sexual pleasure and satisfaction in the previous 4 weeks. The women who used only the pill reported least reduction in sexual pleasure. However, they also reported lower sexual satisfaction than women who used a condom only or pill plus condom. Those using both the pill plus the condom reported the most satisfaction, perhaps because they felt more protected against pregnancy and sexually transmitted disease. This illustrates the psychological effect on contraceptive use and difference between sexual pleasure and sexual satisfaction.[9]

Even though a woman may be sexually depressed by oral contraceptives, there is no evidence that the pill decreases the number of times that she has intercourse if she is married. The failure of the pill to demonstrate decreased frequency of intercourse in married couples might be because it is husbands who usually initiate sexual intercourse.[10]

Because it is the progestin that is the component of a birth control pill that can cause depression, women who want to use the pill, but who get sad, weepy, and apathetic, may try a pill that has a low dose of progestin. Unfortunately, with estrogen alone, breakthrough bleeding often occurs, but even more importantly, high doses of estrogen can increase the risk of blood clot formation that can cause heart attacks.

If you decide to take the pill, there is still a decision to make about which pill. There are many different pills and delivery methods available, with different doses of different kinds of progestin and estrogen. It's nonsense for a woman to feel weepy all the time and to ruin her sex life in order to avoid having a baby. She should try a different pill, or switch to a different method of contraception. If her doctor is not sympathetic, she should switch her doctor, too.

Other Medicines

RU-486
Mifeprex and Korlym are intended to cause abortions within 49 days of gestation. In smaller doses, they have also been used as emergency contraceptives, taken while under the care of a trained healthcare provider. Their active ingredient is a synthetic steroid compound.

PLAN B, NEXT CHOICE
Known as 'morning after pills', they work by a different mechanism than does 'the pill'. They must be taken no later than 72 hours after intercourse, but the closer to the event the better they work. Next Choice requires a second pill 12 hours after the first one. In the spring of 2013, the 'morning after pill' became available over-the-counter and obtainable by anyone, of any age. Their active ingredient is a form of progestin.

NON-PILL OPTIONS

The hormones in 'the pill' can be delivered in other ways, injections or vaginal inserts, to prevent pregnancy. They carry the same risks as does the pill since they deliver the same kind of hormones.

Mirena: An intrauterine device (IUD) that slowly releases a progestin. It may last up to 5 years.

ParaGard: An IUD that releases copper instead of a progestin. A study found no difference between these IUDs on psychological and sexual functioning.[11]

NuvaRing: This works the same way as the combination pills. After insertion into the vagina, it releases both a progestin and estrogen. The ring is removed after 3 weeks. Menstruation occurs and a new ring is inserted after a week.

Depo-Provera: This progestin drug is injected and lasts up to 3 months.

Nexplanon/Implanon NXT or the almost identical **Implanon** is a single-rod contraceptive that is inserted under the skin of a woman's upper arm. The rod contains a type of progestin and lasts up to 3 years.

Nexplanon and **Implanon NXT** are essentially identical to **Implanon** except that **Nexplanon** and **Implanon NXT** have barium sulfate added to make the rod detectable by x-ray.

Part Five
Prescription Meds

9 | Blood Pressure Meds

"Though the doctors treated him, let his blood, and gave him medications to drink, he nevertheless recovered."

– Leo Tolstoy, *War and Peace*

More than 25% of Americans have high blood pressure, also known as hypertension. Although the name implies it, hypertension is not caused by being very tense or stressed. It refers to the tension in the walls of your arteries as your heart pumps blood through your body. If hypertension is not treated, it leads to stroke, kidney damage, heart problems, eye damage, and reduces how long you are likely to live. As you age, you are more likely to high have blood pressure. Unfortunately, blood pressure drugs (antihypertensives) do not cure hypertension. They lower the blood pressure so that it causes limited damage to the body, but once you have it, and you stop taking your drugs, your blood pressure will rise again. If you have had drugs prescribed for hypertension, you will probably need them for the rest of your life. Weight loss, a low salt diet, and a simple diuretic drug that increases your production of urine may lower your blood pressure to normal limits, but only a few persons succeed by only losing weight and changing their diets.

How can you tell if you have it? Blood pressure readings consist of two numbers -- for example, 120 over 80 (written as 120/80 mmHg).

One or both of these numbers can be too high. The top number is called the systolic blood pressure and the bottom number is called the diastolic blood pressure. If your blood pressure numbers are between the normal and the high measures, it is sometimes called pre-hypertension. Your doctor will advise you when either your systolic or diastolic blood pressure is too high for you, based on, for example, your genetics, lifestyle, and other health conditions.

Sexual dysfunction has a major impact on hypertensive patients and their partners.[1] Unfortunately, patients frequently stop taking their blood pressure meds because they think the treatment is worse than the disease.[2] Those with high blood pressure often don't have any symptoms, so they're unhappy to find they're taking drugs that actually make them feel worse or that interfere with their sex lives. Indeed, more men stop taking their blood pressure medicine because they think it has damaged their sexual abilities than for any other reason.

There are six categories of drugs to treat high blood pressure. See Table 9.1 on the next two pages. Because high blood pressure is so common, there are many drug companies that market drug pressure meds and this has resulted in many brand name meds to treat hypertension. There are 74 in this table. Some of the top blood pressure meds are available as generics, so the same drugs are sold under different names. Of the 200 drugs most prescribed in the United States, 16% treat high blood pressure and one of them, the diuretic, hydrochlorothiazide (HCTZ), ranks number 31, 32, 42, 118, and 127 as it also appears in combinations with different brand names.

Table 9.1. High Blood Pressure Prescription Meds	
Common Brand Name	Generic Name
Diuretics	
Midamar	amiloride hydrochloride
Bumex	bumetanide
Hygroton	chlorthalidone
Diuril	chlorothiazide
Lasix	furosemide*
Hydrodiuril, Microzide	HCTZ*
Lozol	indipamide
Mykrox, Zaroxolyn	metazolone
Aldactone	spironolactone
Dyrenium	triamterene*
Moduretic	amiloride hydrochloride + HCTZ*
Aldactazide	spironolactone + HCTZ*
Dyazide, Maxzide	triamterene + HCTZ*
ACE Inhibitors	
Lotensin	benazepril hydrochloride
Captopen	captopril
Vasotec	enalapril*
Monopril	fosinopril sodium
Prinivil, Zestril	lisinopril*
Univasc	moexipril
Aceon	perindopril
Accupril	quinapril hydrochloride
Altace	ramipril
Mavik	trandolapril
Beta-blockers	
Sectral	acebutol
Tenormin	atenolol*
Kerlone	betaxolol
Zebeta	bisoprolol fumarate
Cartrol	carteolol hydrochloride
Coreg	carvedilol*

BLOOD PRESSURE MEDS ▪ 67

Table 9.1. High Blood Pressure Prescription Meds	
Lopressor	metoprolol tartrate*
Toprol-XL	metoprolol succinate*
Corgard	nadolol
Bystolic	nebivolol*
Levatrol	penbutolol sulfate
Visken	pindolol
Inderal	propanolol hydrochloride
Betapace	solotol hydrochloride
Blocadren	timolol maleate
Ziac	bisoprolol + HCTX*
Angiotensin Receptor Blockers (ARBs)	
Atacand	candesartan
Tevetan	eprosartan mesylate
Avapro	irbesartan
Cozaar	losartan potassium
Hyzaar	lisinopril + HCTZ
Micardis	telmisartan
Diovan	valsartan*
Calcium Channel Blockers	
Norvasc, Lortrel	amlodipine besylate*
Vasocor	bepridil
Cardizem, Tiazac	diltiazem hydrochloride
Plendil	felodipine
DynaCirc, DynaCirc CR	isradipine
Cardene	nicardipine
Adalat CC, Procardia XL	nifedipine
Sular	nisoldipine
Calan SR, Covera HS, Isoptin SR, Verelan	verapamil hydrochloride
Central Agonists	
Aldomet	alpha methyldopa
Catapres	clonidine hydrochloride
Wytensin	guanabenz acetate
Tenex	guanfacine hydrochloride

Table 9.1. High Blood Pressure Prescription Meds	
Alpha-blockers	
Alfusozin	alfusozin
Cardura	doxazosin mesylate
Minipress	prazosin hydrochloride
Hytrin	terazosin hydrochloride
Vasodilators	
Apresoline	hydralazine
Loriten	minoxidil

* Among the most frequently prescribed of the top 130 drugs in the U.S. HCTZ is hydrochlorothiazide.

Because of the very large number of meds to treat hypertension, it is not within the scope of this chapter to report on the possible adverse effects on sexual function and other side effects for each drug. For further information see the recommended drug information sites listed in *Chapter 18*. This chapter will, however, report the adverse effects on sexual function for the blood pressure meds in the most frequently prescribed meds in the U.S.

Categories: The categories of drugs treating high blood pressure are known as diuretics, ACE inhibitors, beta-blockers, angiotensin receptor blockers (ARBs), calcium channel blockers, central agonists, and alpha blockers. The older blood pressure meds (diuretics, beta-blockers, central agonists) are most likely to exert negative effects on sexual function, especially erectile dysfunction (ED). The newer meds (calcium channel blockers, ACE inhibitors) have no effect or a beneficial effect.[1]

Although most of the attention has been given to the effect of blood pressure meds on men, women may have their libido depressed by diuretics, beta blockers, and central agonists. There are of course other side effects that are associated with all of these categories. Certain of them, e.g., diarrhea, headache, depression, surely affect sex as they are unlikely to put anyone in the mood for it.

Some drugs that are similar chemically are more likely to cause sex problems than others. As you have seen in Table 9.1, there are many individual and combination drugs to choose from. The variety may make the choice more difficult for the doctor, but it can work to your advantage. If you find you're having problems with erections or ejaculations or libido after taking some of these drugs, and you tell your doctor about it, a switch to a drug that will treat the blood pressure problem and spare the adverse effects on your sex life may be possible.

How do they work?

Diuretics increase the body's output of urine and sodium which tends to relax the blood vessel walls and thus lower the pressure in the arteries. All the drugs in Table 9.1 with "thiazide" at the end of their generic names are diuretics. The thiazides, such as the most commonly prescribed one, hydrochlorothiazide (HCTZ), do not affect sexual function in most persons, but the likelihood increases as people age and up to a third of older men with severe hypertension who are taking a diuretic have problems with impotence.[4] There are also diuretics that do not have "thiazide" at the end of their names but that can also damage sexual functioning. See the table. In addition to erectile dysfunction and depressed libido, some, e.g., spironolactone, can cause breast development in men (gynecomastia), and in women, irregular menses or post-menopausal bleeding.

ACE inhibitors: ACE stands for Angiotensin-converting enzyme. Angiotensin is a chemical that causes the arteries to become narrow, especially in the kidneys but also throughout the body. ACE inhibitors help the body produce less angiotensin, which helps the blood vessels open up, thus lowering blood pressure.

Beta-blockers: Beta-blockers reduce the heart rate and the heart's output of blood, which lowers blood pressure.

Angiotensin receptor blockers (ARBs): These drugs block the effects of the artery narrowing angiotensin. Angiotensin needs a receptor to fit into or bind with in order to constrict the artery. ARBs block the receptors so the angiotensin fails to fit in or bind. This means blood vessels stay open and blood pressure is reduced.

Calcium channel blockers: These prevent calcium from entering the smooth muscle cells of the heart and arteries. When calcium enters these cells, it causes a stronger contraction. By decreasing the calcium, the heart's contraction weakens, which relaxes blood vessels and reduces the heart rate. This results in lower blood pressure.

Central agonists: Central agonists decrease blood vessels' ability to tense up or contract. They follow a different nerve pathway than the alpha and beta-blockers, but achieve the same goal of blood pressure reduction.

Vasodilators: These blood vessel dilators cause the muscle in the walls of the blood vessels (especially the arterioles) to relax, allowing them to widen, which allows the blood to flow through.

Alpha blockers: These relax the muscle tone of the arteries' walls which results in lowered blood pressure.

When a diuretic, such as the mainstay hydrochlorothiazide, together with a low salt diet, do not keep the blood pressure where it ought to be, the doctor will begin adding other drugs that can relax blood vessel walls or reduce the activity of the sympathetic ('fight-or-flight') nervous system. The action of the blood vessels is very important during the arousal phase of the sexual response and the sympathetic nervous system has a prominent role in managing the orgasmic phase. So no surprise, this tells us that a person is almost certain to have sexual difficulties when taking these drugs. Drugs that work best to reduce the blood pressure act directly on the sympathetic nervous system. The more selective they are, the better. Some drugs affect the sympathetic nervous system but they also affect the parasympathetic nervous system and the brain and cause depression. The best high blood pressure fighter would relax only the tiny blood vessels in the arterial blood vessel system, and leave the rest of the body, including the parts needed for sexual activity, including the brain, alone.

Effects on sexual function of high blood pressure meds in the top 130 meds prescribed in the U.S.

Diuretics: all three listed below are associated with impotence and depressed libido.

- Lasix (furosemide)
- Hydrodiuril, Microzide (hydrochlorothiazide)
- Dyrenium (triamterene): rare genital pain

ACE inhibitors: rare (less than 1%) impotence, male breast increase (gynecomastia)

- Vasotec (enalapril)
- Prinivil, Zestril (lisinopril)

Beta-Blockers

- Tenormin (atenolol): in women depressed libido
- Bystolic (nebivolol): none reported
- Coreg (carvedilol): none reported
- Lopressor (metoprolol tartrate): in women rare depressed libido
- Toprol-XL (metoprolol succinate): none reported

ARBs

- Diovan (valsartan): impotence less than 0.2%

Calcium channel blockers

- Norvasc, Lortrel (amlodipine besylate): male and female depressed libido

The Beta-blockers, metoprolols (Lopressor, Toprol-XL), are more selective about where they work in the body than some of the other antihypertensives. They block the action of chemical messengers at certain kinds of receptors in the sympathetic nervous system. That's why, if you're taking one of them, you might hear your doctor say the words, "beta-adrenergic blocking agent." The meaning to you is a drug that is less likely than most others to interfere with libido and potency. Studies of beta-blockers bisoprolol, carvedilol, and nebivolol, found no worsening of sexual function in hypertensives.[5]

One of the ARBs, Cozaar (losartan) was tested in diabetic men. When given with the male performance enhancer, Cialis (tadalafil), it was more effective in treating ED than either drug alone.[6] Also, in another study it reduced symptoms of androgen deficiency and did not contribute to ED.[7] Plendil (felodipine), a calcium channel blocker, with an ARB, Avapro (irbesartan) was found more effective in treating hypertensive men with mild ED than felodipine and metoprolol.[8] Moreover, felopidine plus irbesartan reduced blood pressure equally as did metoprolol but the combination improved sexual function more in young and middle-aged women with hypertension.[9]

Lozol (indapamide) decreased the risk of worsening sexual function in men with uncontrolled hypertension.[10]

The **Central Agonists** are blood pressure meds that are no longer among the most frequently prescribed, probably because they were associated with the most sexual dysfunction. Two of them, for example, Aldomet (methyldopa) and Catapres (clonidine) are associated with impotence, delayed ejaculation, breast enlargement, lactation, depressed libido, and menstruation irregularities.[11-15]

Unfortunately few Clinical Practice Guidelines (CPGs) were found to emphasize the importance of assessing sexual function prior to initiation or follow-up of antihypertensive therapy in a literature search of the World Wide Web, bibliographies of retrieved guidelines, and official home pages of major medical societies.[16] Only a minority of

CPGs for the treatment of hypertension considered ED or other sexual issues as either an adverse outcome or as a factor to consider in treatment. Certainly, finding the right blood-pressure drug or combination can be a complicated problem, and depends on many factors other than sexual. Some drugs can't be used because of other health problems that would be exacerbated by the drug's action. If this is the case, your doctor or pharmacist should be able to tell you about it. Don't make a discussion of the damaging effects of an antihypertensive drug on your sex life a topic with yourself, your neighbor, or your spouse alone. What can they do? Do yourself a favor. Tell the doctor or pharmacist. The two of you can then decide what to do about it. The good news is that there are more blood pressure meds that do not cause sexual dysfunction than there used to be and some that may even help.

10

Cholesterol Lowering Meds

"... with regard to disease .... do good or [at least] do no harm."

– Hippocrates

Statins are among the most prescribed drugs in the U.S. due to their effectiveness in decreasing cholesterol levels in the blood. Fibrates also lower cholesterol, and in addition triglycerides, but they are not prescribed as often as statins because they are usually reserved for patients who can't take statins or who have unusually high cholesterol levels.

Statin Prescription Drugs *	
Brand Name	**Generic Name**
Lipitor, Torvast	atorvastatin**
Lescol, Lescol XL	fluvastatin
Altocor, Altoprev, Mevacor	lovastatin**
Compactin	mevastatin
Livalo, Pitava	pitavastatin
Lipostat, Pravachol, Selektine	pravastatin**
Crestor	rosuvastatin**
Lipex, Zocor	simvastatin**
Caduet	atorvastatin & amlodipine

Statin Prescription Drugs *	
Advicor	lovastatin & niacin
Vytorin	simvastatin & ezetimide**
Simcor	simvastatin & niacin
Juvisync	simvastatin & sitagliptin
Fibrate Prescription Drugs*	
Bezalip	bezafibrate
Modalim	ciprofibrate
TriCor	fenofibrate**
Trilipix	fenofibric acid
Lopid	gemfibrozil

* Most statins and fibrates are available generically and may have more than one brand name.

** One of the top prescription drugs in the U.S. in 2012.

And do the statins and/or the fibrates adversely affect sexual function? The evidence suggests that yes they do, with fibrates more likely although the risk is low. However, given the very large number of prescriptions written for them, especially the statins, even a low risk means that the number of users is significant. Both kinds can cause impotence and difficulty in achieving orgasm for both men and women.

Given the benefit of the statins and fibrates in preventing strokes and heart attacks, should you stop taking them to avoid rare, but possible, impotence or loss of libido? The answer is probably no because you can probably eliminate the problem by switching to a different one. You tell your prescribing physician about the problem and ask for a change.

Surprisingly, statins not only carry the rare risk of affecting sexual function adversely, they are also used to treat impotence in some cases. Let's look at the research. When might they adversely affect sexual function, when might they help sexual function, and when are the effects uncertain?

Adverse effects. A review of randomized clinical trials and studies with other research designs supported the existence of statin-associated adverse effects including sexual dysfunction.[1]

Another systematic review of studies in computerized databases and Internet sources of almost all of the statins and fibrates on the market concluded that both might cause impotence.[2]

Another study funded by the government found that both statin-taking men and women reported increased difficulty achieving orgasm. Yes, their LDL cholesterol levels decreased, but so did their levels of sexual pleasure.[1,3]

What causes the adverse effects on sexual function to happen? It turns out that cholesterol is a building-block of testosterone, estrogens, and other sex hormones in the body. So it follows that, when the statins and fibrates do their job and decrease cholesterol, the decrease in cholesterol also decreases the hormones that facilitate sexual functioning.

Not surprisingly, some preexisting health conditions can increase the risk of erectile dysfunction (ED) after statins are taken. Patients with risk factors for heart disease, including age, smoking, and diabetes, were found in one study to be more likely to develop ED after statin therapy than they were before it.[4]

When might statins and/or fibrates help sexual dysfunction? Several studies have reported that statin therapy has helped men with ED. One of the most recent, recruited 173 men who were not being treated for ED and randomized them to simvastatin (Zocor) or placebo once daily for six months. At the end of the six months there was no significant difference in their erectile function score, but there was a small (5% vs. 2%) significant improvement in their reported ED-specific Quality of Life (MED-QoL) score.[5]

Another study compared the effect on ED of atorvastatin (Lipitor) to regular tadalafil (Cialis) use. Although the statin alone improved ED, particularly in men with very high cholesterol, Cialis three times a week was significantly better than the statin alone.[6]

Statin therapy may help men recover their erectile function more quickly after nerve-sparing prostate surgery[7] and atorvastatin (Lipitor) may increase the effect of sildenafil (Viagra) in men who have not responded to Viagra alone.[8,9]

Any disagreement? Yes, there is disagreement relative to the effect of one of the most frequently prescribed statins, Zocor (simvastatin), in patients with ED caused by endothelial dysfunction. Endothelial dysfunction is associated with most forms of cardiovascular disease, such as hypertension, coronary artery disease, chronic heart failure, peripheral artery disease, diabetes, and kidney failure. Men with ED caused by endothelial dysfunction were randomized to receive simvastatin or a placebo for 6 months and then one of the male performance enhancers (Levitra) to take on demand for the next 4 months. There was a significant reduction in cholesterol in the group with the statin but no difference in ED in either the placebo or the statin group. The researchers concluded that their study did not support the use of simvastatin for ED.[10] In addition, *Health News* from NHS Choices stated in its April 2013 *Behind the Headlines* release, that atorvastatin (Lipitor) given to men for whom sildenafil (Viagra) had not worked,"helped improve symptoms of erectile dysfunction, but not to such an extent that it could be considered an effective treatment."

It's clear that ED is common, is variable in severity, and has many causes. It behooves men who have it and want to improve their sex lives, to explore the possible reasons they have it or are getting it, and the possible fixes with their physicians.

11

Antidepressants

"Tell us please, what treatment in an emergency is administered by ear?".... I met his gaze and I did not blink. "Words of comfort," I said to my father."

– Abraham Verghese, *Cutting for Stone*

Between 30% and 70% of people diagnosed with depression experience sexual dysfunction. Alas, many of the antidepressants they take to treat their depression can also cause sex problems, which can begin as soon as the first week after starting them. Almost any kind of sex problem can occur. In men, they frequently cause erectile dysfunction (ED) and in women, vaginal dryness, decreased genital sensation, and menstruation disorders. In both men and women, decreased libido and difficulty in achieving orgasm occur.[1]

Because sex problems can produce psychological distress and decreased self-esteem, many people stop taking their antidepressant drug when they happen. Fortunately, there are now antidepressants that can improve your mental state with less chance of causing those unwanted sex problems.[2] Not only that, some of them actually help premature ejaculation (PE), a problem that occurs in more men (as many as one-third more) than erectile dysfunction.[3,4]

There are nine kinds of prescription meds used to treat depression. In the U.S. they account for 50 or more antidepressants with different brand names. Nine of these are among the top 130 meds prescribed in the U.S. See the drugs starred in the tables below.

Selective serotonin reuptake inhibitors (SSRIs) are thought to moderate the neurotransmitter serotonin in the brain. Because serotonin moderates a sense of self-control and well-being, it is believed that too little of it in the brain causes depression. However, there is no way to measure it in the brain so it's a theory, not a scientific fact. The theory also holds that too much of it overwhelms the neurotransmitter dopamine which says, 'Let's have sex' and instead sends the message 'Forget about it' and that's why the SSRIs may decrease depression but also affect sex adversely. SSRIs, however, are an old and frequent treatment for premature ejaculation (PE).[5] Dapoxetine (Priligy), an SSRI originally developed to treat depression was found to be eliminated by the body too fast to treat depression, but this made it suitable to treat PE.[6]

SSRI Antidepressants	
Brand Names	Generic Names
Celexa	citalopram*
Priligy	dapoxetine
Lexapro, Cipralex	escitalopram*
Paxil, Seroxat	paroxetine*
Prozac	fluoxetine*
Luvox	fluvoxamine
Zoloft, Lustral	sertraline*

*   Among top 130 prescribed drugs in the U.S.

Selective norepinephrine reuptake inhibitors (SNRIs) inhibit the absorption (reuptake) of norepinephrine. Serotonin has played the major role in how to treat depression but norepinephrine is now a player. The recent development of the SNRI reboxetine, facilitated clinical investigation of the role of the noradrenergic system in different aspects of depression. It was found to be at least as effective as the

SSRIs in treating depression and to cause less nausea and less sexual dysfunction.

SNRI Antidepressants	
Brand Names	**Generic Names**
Strattera	atomoxetine
Edronax	reboxetine
Vivalan	viloxazine

Noradrenergic and specific serotonergic antidepressants (NaSSAs) inhibit the reuptake of serotonin and noradrenaline. They therefore act the same as the SSRIs but the noradrenergic action helps prevent the side effects often associated with the SSRI antidepressants. Mirtazapine was compared with tricyclic antidepressants in 29 clinical trials and found to work as well but cause less sexual dysfunction.[7] Another study concluded it was a good choice for the treatment of SSRI-caused sexual dysfunction.[8] It has also been suggested that it be combined with other antidepressants to shorten the time until their antidepressants effect kicks in and lessens their sexual dysfunction effect.[9]

NaSSA Antidepressants	
Brand Names	**Generic Names**
Tolvan	mianserin
Remeron, Avanza, Zispin	mirtazapine

Serotonin-norepinephrine reuptake inhibitors (SNRIs) ease depression by changing the levels of neurotransmitters which communicate among brain cells. They block the absorption (reuptake) of the neurotransmitters serotonin and norepinephrine. They also affect certain other neurotransmitters. Changing the balance of these chemicals seems to help brain cells send and receive messages, which in turn boosts mood. All SNRIs generally cause similar side effects which can include sexual problems, such as reduced desire, difficulty reaching orgasm, and erectile dysfunction.

SNRI Antidepressants	
Brand Names	Generic Names
Pristiq	desfenlafaxine
Cymbalta	duloxetine*
Ixel, Savella	milnacipran
Effexor	venlafaxine*
Fetzima	levomilnacipran

*   Among top 130 prescribed drugs in the U.S.

Serotonin antagonist and reuptake inhibitors (SARIs) antidepressants act by inhibiting the absorption of serotonin, norepinephrine, and dopamine in the brain, but not as selectively as do the SSRIs. They are prescribed for major depressive disorder. Trazodone (Desyrel), for example, one of the most frequently prescribed antidepressants, rarely causes priapism but has been associated with sexual dysfunction, however less frequently than the SSRIs.[10,11]

SARI Antidepressants	
Brand Names	Generic Names
Axiomin, Etonin	etoperidone
Normarex	lorpiprazole
YM-992, YM-35995	lubazadone
Psigodal	mepiprazole
Serzone, Nefadar	nefazodone
Desyrel	trazodone*
Brintellix	vortioxetine

*   Among top 130 prescribed drugs in the U.S.

Norepinephrine-dopamine reuptake inhibitors (NDRIs) act by blocking the neurotransmitters norepinephrine and dopamine. This leads to increased concentrations of both norepinephrine and dopamine in the brain. **Norepinephrine and dopamine disinhibitors** (**NDDIs**) act at specific sites to disinhibit downstream norepinephrine and dopamine release in the brain. Change in libido is a possible side effect.

Bupropion (Wellbutrin, Zyban) has been found as effective an antidepressant as some tricyclic and SSRI antidepressants, but associated with less sexual dysfunction than the SSRI, escitalopram (Lexapro, Cipralex).[12]

NDRI and NDDI Antidepressants	
Brand Names	Generic Names
Wellbutrin, Zyban	bupropion
Valdoxan, Melitor, Thymanax	agomelatine

Monoamine Oxidase Antidepressants (MAOIs) inhibit the enzyme which breaks down the neurotransmitters dopamine, serotonin, and norepinephrine in the brain. The newer ones are the last two in the table below. As there are potentially fatal interactions between older MAOIs and certain foods and other drugs, the irreversible MAOIs are rarely prescribed except for selegiline (Eldypryl, Emsam) which is a patch form. Because it bypasses the stomach, it has less propensity to cause harm.[13]

MAOIs may cause impotence and delay of ejaculation.[13,15] Some, phenelzine (Nardil) and tranylcypromine (Parnate), may also cause ED. However, there are also reports of some of these drugs causing an increase in libido and on rare occasions hypersexuality. In one private medical experiment, six normal men volunteered to take Parnate. After one week, three of the six reported changes in their sex response. One became temporarily impotent. One reported he had an increase in his sex drive, and the third said he was so stimulated he was embarrassed by his uncontrollable erections.[16]

In one of the few reports of a drug affecting female sexual response, an adverse effect of Nardil was found by accident. Seven patients, three men and four women, were given Nardil to treat narcolepsy, a rare illness causing extreme sleepiness. However, after taking the drug, all three of the men reported they were awake but had problems achieving an erection. Two of the four women said they couldn't achieve orgasms anymore.[17]

Monoamine Antidepressants (MAOIs)	
Brand Names	**Generic Names**
Marplan	isocarboxazid
Nardil	phenelzine
Eldepryl, Emsam	selegiline
Parnate	tranylcypromine
Aurorix, Manerix	moclobemide
Pirazidol	pirlindol

Tricyclic Antidepressants typically block the absorption of norepinephrine and serotonin in the brain. There are more reports of the effects of the tricyclic antidepressants on libido and sexual performance than there are of the MAOIs.[18-20] The tricyclics alter the nerve-hormone chemistry in the central nervous system and this change affects the neurotransmitters. As was noted with the MAOIs, when this interference occurs, sexual function, and particularly the orgasm phase, may be disturbed.

Amitriptyline (Elavil, Endep) was introduced in the U.S. more than 50 years ago but is still regularly prescribed for depression. While it works well, in a review of 39 clinical trials which included 3509 subjects, more subjects withdrew due to its side effects, which included sexual dysfunction, than those on placebos.[21]

Imipramine (Tofranil) is one of the oldest and most common tricyclic antidepressants in use. In one study, imipramine was given to 107 men and 198 women, of whom a third had depression, and the rest other mental problems. Imipramine depressed the sexual functioning in six percent of the patients, and stimulated it in about two percent. The stimulation was believed by the physician running the study to be a secondary effect following from the improvement in mood that is the primary effect of the drug.[18] In another study, six normal men were given imipramine. After one week the drug affected the sexual function of three of the men. One man experienced a decrease in his sexual drive that eventually led to impotence. A second could not achieve an erection, and a third had a decrease in his libido.[16] Partly because of the adverse effects of imipramine on sexual function, physicians began to try other tricyclic antidepressants, especially amitriptyline (Elavil), to treat depression and symptoms of anxiety. There are reports of protriptyline (Vivactil) causing sexual problems, but fewer than for amytriptyline and protriptyline.[16]

The official labeling of clomipramine (Anafranil) cautions that side effects include impotence, ejaculation failure, decreased libido, and menstrual and breast disorders. However, clomipramine is an effective drug to treat PE.[3,22] and tianeptine (Stablon, Coaxil, Tatinol) is an effective therapy for treating depression and ED.[23]

Tricyclic Antidepressants	
Brand Names	**Generic Names**
Elavil, Endep	amitriptyline*
Anafranil	clomipramine
Adapin, Sinequan	doxepin
Tofranil	imipramine
Surmontil	trimipramine
Norpramin	desipramine
Pamelor, Avantyl, Noritren	nortriptyline
Vivactil	protriptyline
Stablon, Coaxil, Tatinol	tianeptine
Servector	amineptine
Insidon, Pramolan, Ensidon, Oprimol	opipramol

* Among top 130 prescribed drugs in the U.S.

Don't give up. In one study of sixty male patients on antidepressants, only three of the men volunteered that they were experiencing a sexual problem, although about twenty of the men admitted it when they were asked directly.[16] In another study, 42% of men on antidepressants simply waited for the problem to go away.[24] Not all doctors will ask, so it is important for patients to know that if they inform their doctor, the dose of the antidepressant may be decreased, or they may be switched to a different drug which can treat the medical problem without causing an adverse effect on libido or sexual performance.[2] The antidepressants are not all alike, nor are patients. A drug that causes a problem in one patient will not necessarily cause it in another, even at the same dose. One of the drugs in the antidepressant group may cause a problem and another may not, even though the two drugs are very similar in chemical structure. There are antidepressant drugs to treat premature ejaculation but many doctors don't inquire about it and many patients don't volunteer or admit they have PE.[4]

Talking to their doctor about their sexual feelings and response may be particularly important for women. About 50% of women are considered to be depressed when they are menopausal, and many doctors give them antidepressants.[25,26] Because there is so little in the medical literature about the effect of the antidepressants on women's sexual function, physicians may be less likely to expect an adverse effect, or may associate a sexual change with the woman's depression or her age rather than the drug. However, there is no reason to believe that this group of drugs works any differently in women than it does in men, or that sexual dysfunction should happen any less often in women than men.

Patients should know that antidepressants are powerful and important drugs which can help them function better at work and at home if they are suffering from depression. The experience of an adverse effect on their sexual function, which occurs in up to 30% of patients, depending on the particular antidepressant, should not cause them to discontinue taking a drug altogether, but to request that the dose be reduced or that a different antidepressant be tried.

12

Minor Tranquilizers and Anti-Anxiety Meds

"Man is not worried by real problems so much as by his imagined anxieties about real problems."

– Epictetus

Minor tranquilizers are listed in the table below. Because they have been marketed for so many years, most are available generically and have many brand names. For example, Valium (diazepam), the second minor tranquilizer on the market, is now sold with more than 500 other brand names around the world. For this reason, not all brand names are listed in the table.

Minor Tranquilizers and Anti-Anxiety Meds	
Most Common Brand Names	**Generic Names**
Xanax (and many others)	alprazolam*
Buspar	buspirone
Librium (and many others)	chlordiazapoxide
Tranxene	clorazepate
Klonopin	clonazepam
Valium (and many others)	diazepam*
Dalmane	flurazepam
Eurodin, ProSom	estazolam
Verstran	lorazepam*

Minor Tranquilizers and Anti-Anxiety Meds	
Equanil, Miltown	meprobamate
Dormicum, Hypnovel, Versed	midazolam
Mogadon (and many others)	nitrazepam
Serax (and many others)	oxazepam
Ativan (and many others)	prazepam
Doral, Dormalin	quazepam
Restoril, Normison	temazepam
Halcion (and many others)	triazolam

* Among top 130 prescribed drugs in the U.S.

The major tranquilizers are anti-psychotic drugs. You will find them in *Chapter 13*. The minor tranquilizers generally relieve anxiety and are also known as anti-anxiety meds. They may also, in some people, induce a loss of inhibition and a feeling of well-being. And they may also cause sexual dysfunction. All but two of them in the table, Buspar (buspirone) and Equanil or Miltown (meprobamate), are benzodiazepines.

How Do They Work?

No one is absolutely sure, but the most prevalent theory is that benzodiazepines increase the effect of a neurotransmitter, gamma-amiobutyric acid (GABA), in the brain. That results in sedative, sleep inducing, anti-anxiety, anticonvulsant, and muscle relaxing effects.[1,2]

Benzodiazepines are classed as short, intermediate, or long-acting. The short and intermediate ones are preferred for insomnia; the longer-acting for anxiety.[3] There is a long list of possible side-effects associated with the minor tranquilizers.

Although millions of persons take minor tranquilizers and three of them are among the most frequently prescribed drugs in the U.S., reports of them causing a problem with sexual function are rare and if reported, usually in less than 4% of users. You probably shouldn't be concerned that they will affect your sexual function, but it's not impossible. Of course side effects are more likely with large doses.

A benzodiazepine not on the table is flunitrazepine whose street name is "date rape drug". It is no longer a legal drug in the U.S.

Among the list of possible effects on sex are changes in sexual desire.[4] Other sexual dysfunction effects include menstruation irregularities, breast pain, vaginal dryness, impotence and trouble reaching orgasm. The decrease in libido is believed to result indirectly from the psychological depression sometimes caused by tranquilizers.[5] For example, one man, after taking a large dose of Librium (chlordiazepoxide), told his doctor that Librium caused him to have difficulty with ejaculation. That prolonged the duration of his sexual intercourse and sometimes he couldn't ejaculate at all. When he stopped taking Librium, his difficulty with ejaculation disappeared.[6] On the other hand, there are very rare reports of increased libido after taking Xanax (alprazolam).

On a positive note, the ability of the minor tranquilizers to reduce anxiety and stress may make sexual relations so much more relaxed and pleasurable for you that you interpret your feelings as increased sexual desire. On the other hand, you can't enjoy sex very much if you're so tranquilized you're asleep.

13

Antipsychotics

"Mental illness is so much more complicated than any pill that any mortal could invent."

— Elizabeth Wurtzel

Although antipsychotics, as a name for a group of drugs, suggest they are only prescribed for deeply disturbed persons, this is by no means the case. They are also prescribed for thousands of people with only minor psychological issues and for many nursing home residents, where they act as major tranquilizers. Many of them cause sexual dysfunction in both sexes. Loss of sexual function may not disturb most people in nursing homes very much, but loss of your sexual function may well disturb you. There is quite a difference among the antipsychotics with regard to their potential for affecting sexual behavior, so if you are taking one of these drugs now, are living with someone taking one, or may be taking one in the future, you'll want to know which ones are the biggest troublemakers.

Common Brand Names*	Generic Names
Abilify, Aripiprex	aripiprazole
Thorazine	chlorpromazine
Sordinol	clopenthixol
Clozaril, Fazaclo	clozapine
Modecate	fluphenazine

Common Brand Names*	Generic Names
Imap, Redeptin	fluspirilene
Haldol	haloperidol
Adasuve, Loxapac, Loxitane	loxapine
Zyprexa	olanzapine
Invega Sustenna	paliperidone palmitate
Semap, Micefal	penfluridol
Peragal, Perazin, Pernazinum, Taxilen	perazine
Trilafon	perphenazine
Compro, ProComp	prochlorperazine
Pentazine, Phenergan	promethazine
Seroquel, Ketipinor, Xeroquel	quetiapine
Risperdal	risperidone
Serdolect, Serlect	sertindole
Stelazine	trifluoperazine
Navane, Thixit	tiotixene
Geodon, Zeldox	ziprasidone

* Other generic versions with different brand names may be available.

A word of caution. Antipsychotic drugs are major tranquilizers. They are primarily prescribed to treat delusions, hallucinations, bipolar disorder, and most often for schizophrenia. They are also prescribed for alcoholism, aggressiveness, severe depression, and lack of impulse control. The antipsychotics should be reserved for serious psychological disturbances, such as schizophrenia, and not for minor depression, insomnia, or anxiety. The minor tranquilizers and antidepressants are better for these problems. Indeed, the side effects of antipsychotics on sexual function seem as likely to cause depression and anxiety as to alleviate them.

The medical literature includes many reviews of the relationship of antipsychotics to sexual dysfunction.[1-11] A large number of antipsychotics adversely affect sexual function in one or more areas: libido, arousal, and orgasm. However, symptoms have been reported related to penile erection, priapism, lubrication, orgasm, ejaculation, menstruation, breast pain, milk production, and overall sexual satisfaction. Two conclusions one can draw from the reviews is that more information is needed primarily because of the high numbers of subjects who quit before the end of clinical trials and poor study design.[5] Sexual dysfunction is a major reason patients stop taking their meds and withdraw from clinical trials.[1,2]

Studies have found that antipsychotics cause more sexual dysfunction in men than women:[7,12-15] for example, in one study 59% of men and 49% of women with schizophrenia.[15] It's probably not news to you that women's brains are different than men's. Thus no surprise that the antipsychotics would affect the sex differences in the brains of men and women who have schizophrenia differently. Some efforts have been made to address the differences in sexual dysfunction caused by antipsychotics with hormones such as estrogen and testosterone, but the jury is still out.[12]

The first generation of antipsychotics, referred to often as "typical" antipsychotics, were produced in the 1950s. The oldest and most common ones still in use are chlorpromazine (Thorazine) and haloperidol (Haldol). Most of the second generation antipsychotics, now known as "atypical" antipsychotics, have been developed more recently and one of the reasons was to decrease the sexual dysfunction caused by the first generation ("typicals") of these drugs. They are now considered the front line of antipsychotics. The "atypical" ones include aripiprazole, clozapine, olanzapine, quetiapine, risperidone, and sertindole.[5]

How do antipsychotics cause sexual dysfunction? Antipsychotics block the effects of dopamine in the brain and that in turn stimulates the pituitary gland to increase prolactin. And that increase of prolactin causes sexual dysfunction. The second generation ("atypical") antipsychotics are less likely than the "typical" ones to increase prolactin and are thus less likely to cause sexual dysfunction.[4]

Can the sexual dysfunction effects of antipsychotics be fixed? Fix strategies include dose reduction, drug holidays, add another med, and switch the med.[2] There is very little research in this area and what there is, has mostly been done in male patients taking antipsychotics for schizophrenia. One review of research studies reported that adding sildenafil (Viagra) increased the duration of erections and increased sexual intercourse satisfaction. Adding a drug that treats Parkinson's Disease had no effect. Switching to the "atypical" quetiapine (Seroquel, Ketipinor, Xeroquel), from risperidone (Risperdal) did not help, but switching from risperidone to olanzapine (Zyprexa) did improve sexual functioning.[2] Another review concluded that adding sildenafil (Viagra) or aripiprazole (Ablify, Aripiprex) improved sexual dysfunction but adding two other meds did not.[3] This review also reported that quetiapine helped in two studies but in a third did not help.

Aripiprazole (Ablify, Aripiprex): In a randomized clinical trial, the group receiving aripripazole had less sexual dysfunction than three other atypical antipsychotics (olanzapine, quetiapine, risperidone).[16] In another study, aripripazole was taken by both men and women, and both symptoms of psychosis and sexual dysfunction were improved but with faster improvement in the men than in the women. The most notable improvement was in delayed ejaculation and orgasm.[17]

Olanzapine (Zyprexa): Olanzapine produced fewer adverse side effects in patients with schizophrenia than did risperidone in a number of studies, including those that switched patients to this "atypical" medication from risperidone (Risperdal) or one of the "typical" antipsychotics.[2,5]

Paliperadone palmitate (Invega Sustenna): Whereas this injected med is more effective than a placebo, studies have found it no more effective and with no fewer effects on sexual functioning than risperidone (Risperdal).[4] Priapism may occur, but in less than 1% of men taking it.[18]

Risperadone (Risperdal): Other "atypical" antipsychotics have the same or fewer adverse effects on sexual functioning than this med which may decrease libido and produce unwanted breast milk.[2,5]

Sertindole (Serdolect, Serlect): Two studies comparing this med with risperidone (Risperdal) in men with schizophrenia, concluded sertindole may cause more sexual dysfunction, specifically decreased libido.[5,18]

Ziprasidone (Geodon, Zeldox): This med may cause priapism, but in fewer than one percent of men.[18]

Summary: The antipsychotics are very powerful, many with serious side effects that can be permanent, but their adverse effect on sexual functioning is usually temporary. The newer "atypical" antipsychotics have fewer adverse effects than the older "typical" ones. Health care professionals often are unaware of the sexual problems that negatively impact their patients' satisfaction with treatment, quality of life, and compliance with their meds.[19] So, patients on antipsychotics or their caregivers are urged to speak up. There are fixes.

14

And a Few Others

"We strive for error-free medicine in a world that is sometimes all too human."

– Michael Burgess

Chemo

All drugs are chemicals, but cancer-fighting drugs are commonly referred to as "chemo", short for "chemotherapy", in contrast with other kinds of treatment, especially radiation. Drugs used to treat cancer (also called antineoplastics) often decrease fertility. Sometimes patients take four or more different kinds at the same time. Chemo almost always has other unpleasant side effects too. Hair loss is a prime example, but because the cancers being treated are often life-threatening, most cancer patients willingly suffer the side effects in exchange for a chance to survive.

Antineoplastics do not affect men's desire, but they do cause them to have a low sperm count or no sperm at all. About half of men return to normal in from two to seven years after taking the drugs, and about half continue to have low sperm counts.[1] Young women given chemo for leukemia before puberty usually don't have any fertility problems, but there can be problems if given after puberty.[2]

Fungus Meds

Nizoral (ketoconazole) is given topically and orally as a tablet for fungus infections. Its official FDA labeling cautions that it can cause impotence, gynecomastia (excessive development of male breasts), and oligospermia (sperm deficiency). It works via two mechanisms. First, and most notably, high oral doses block both testicular and adrenal androgen biosynthesis, which leads to a reduction in circulating testosterone levels.[3] Second, although a weak effect, Nizoral is an androgen receptor antagonist, so it competes with androgens such as testosterone.[4]

Irregular Heart Beats

Norpace (disopyramide) is a drug that treats the kind of irregular heartbeats that may predispose to heart attacks. The drug works by interfering with a chemical messenger in the parasympathetic nervous system. Most drugs aren't very selective and this is no exception. It also interferes with chemical messengers responsible for erection, so that a man on this drug may have sexual desire but be unable to perform.[5]

Ulcer Meds

Tagamet (cimetidine) has been touted as a miracle drug for persons with gastric ulcers, but it's not so great for fertility. Doctors found that sperm production was decreased more than 40% in men who took this drug for nine weeks, and it has also caused gynecomastia (male breast development). The level of testosterone in the blood is not decreased by cimetidine. Thus, the effect on the sperm-producing tissues is probably direct.[6] Obviously, caution is advised when Tagamet is given to young men for prolonged time periods, and regular sperm counts should be taken.

Part Six
Nonmedical Med Use

15

Legal Meds Used for Nonmedical Purposes: Can They Affect Your Sex Life?

"Medicine sometimes snatches away health, sometimes gives it."

– Ovid

Almost everyone would love to find a pill or potion that would make sex more exciting, that would make the objects of our desire find us as irresistible as we find them, that would make men into inexhaustible lovers and guarantee women multiple orgasms. Imagine a pill that would raise us to new pleasure heights and promise that nobody had it better than we did. What wouldn't many of us give for that?

When drugs are used medically, that is prescribed by doctors, to correct sexual problems, few people would deny them to anyone. However, when drugs are used in relationship to sex for nonmedical reasons, it seems there are still some very strong anti-pleasure values around, and that many people disapprove of anyone using a drug for no other reason than to increase sexual desire or pleasure. However, despite the disapproval of many, legal drugs are used nonmedically to increase sexual desire and to expand or modify the actual sexual experience, sometimes through changing states of consciousness.

In addition, legal drugs are used for nonmedical reasons to build muscle, to stay awake, and to experience euphoria.

A Note on Nonlegal Drugs

The Drug Enforcement Administration (DEA) of the U.S. classifies drugs in five categories primarily according to their potential for causing addiction or dependence but also when used for nonmedical purposes. No prescriptions may be written for Schedule I substances as they are considered to have no currently accepted medical use in the United States and they lack an accepted safety level for use even under medical supervision. There are, however, several instances when a substance listed on Schedule I, such as one of marijuana's active ingredients, a cannabinoid, is also listed in Schedule III for a limited use. As the potential for abuse increases, the Schedule rank decreases, e.g., from 3 to 2, and affects the amount of control, which includes rules about refills and record keeping. Schedule V includes the over-the-counter drugs (OTCs), but still are required to have a medical purpose. Historically, the tendency has been for the DEA to move substances to lower rank numbers thus making them less available.

This chapter includes the use and effects on sexual function of uppers, downers, marijuana, narcotics (a term that technically includes all non-legal substances, but is often used to refer to morphine-like drugs), inhalants, and anabolic steroids.

Uppers: Cocaine and Amphetamines

Cocaine and amphetamines (plural, since there are many) are substances whose use has become more restricted by the DEA over time and both reportedly affect sexual function. The how, or what, what form, and how much are the questions.

Cocaine has moved from the "upper" in a bottle of Coca-Cola to a Schedule II drug with its only legal use as a topical anesthetic. Cocaine varies from a leaf of the plant, *Erythroxylon coca*, chewed daily in Peru and served to tourists as a welcome tea in hotels, to lines snorted in the U.S. by guests at parties and referred to by street names such as "snow" and "happy dust".

The topical use of cocaine recreationally is relatively rare. Most "coke" is sniffed because it is absorbed quite rapidly through the mucous membranes of the nose. Swallowing is the slowest route; smoking is faster than sniffing, but wasteful, and injecting is the quickest way to get "hit."

Amphetamines, the first of which, Benzedrine, came on the market in 1932, were prescribed for fatigue, heroin addiction, and appetite suppression. They were originally on Schedule III, but were moved to Schedule II in 1971.

Despite their different routes of ingestion (cocaine is commonly "snorted" while amphetamines are swallowed or injected), the physiological effects of cocaine and amphetamines are very similar. Moreover, they resemble, in an exaggerated way, their more pedestrian cousin, caffeine.

The 1965 edition of the most widely used pharmacology textbook, Goodman and Gilman's *The Pharmacologic Basis of Therapeutics*, said of cocaine: "The subjective effects of cocaine include an elevation of mood that often reaches proportions of euphoric excitement. It produces a marked decrease in hunger, an indifference to pain, and is reported to be the most potent anti-fatigue agent known. The user enjoys a feeling of great muscular strength and increased mental capacity." A more recent edition of Goodman and Gilman said of amphetamine: "The main results . . . are as follows: wakefulness, alertness, and a decreased sense of fatigue; elevation of mood, with increased initiative, confidence, and ability to concentrate; often elation and euphoria; increase in motor and speech activity. Performance of only simple mental tasks is improved. . . . Physical performance, for example, in athletics, is improved." It appears that if one paragraph were exchanged for the other, few would notice the difference.

There were no investigations into the effects of amphetamines and cocaine on sexual function reported in the leading medical journals from 2003-2013, except as incidental to multiple drug use or risky sex behavior. However, people who have come to drug clinics and programs have been questioned. Their reports are purely subjective and in many cases are questionable because other drugs, especially alcohol and marijuana, were used concomitantly.

Despite the lack of research, it can be said that cocaine does not cause anyone to engage in a sexual act or to have a spontaneous sexual response. It only modifies sexual activity and perceptions of it. If there is a value for abstention in the society in which it is used, cocaine will exert its pharmacological effects of central nervous system stimulation and appetite suppression, but it will not act as a sexual stimulant. If the societal values permit or encourage full sexual satisfaction and exploration, cocaine's stimulant effects will make people feel and respond differently during sexual activity, just as it does during other activities.

The difference of cocaine from amphetamine in terms of its effects is that cocaine is a very strong local or topical anesthetic that has a pronounced numbing effect on the eyes, the gums, the inside of the nose, and other mucous membranes. For this reason, cocaine is sometimes applied to the glans of the penis. If men have a problem with premature ejaculation or merely want to have intercourse for a longer time than is usually possible, a little cocaine applied topically desensitizes and delays the time to reach ejaculation. Similarly, women may apply cocaine to the clitoris and genital mucosa or take a very expensive cocaine douche so they can have intercourse for a longer time.

Currently the following amphetamines are on the market - they all are dextroamphetamine or metabolize into it in the body: Adderall, Benzedrine, Dexedrine, Dextroamphet, Dextrostat, Didrex, ProCentra, and Vyvanse. The injectable amphetamines, Desoxyn and Methedrine (methamphetamine), are no longer legally available. There are more than a dozen street names for dextroamphetamine with "speed" probably the most common.

A number of amphetamine related stimulant drugs are also on the market, some used mostly for weight control and others for hyperactivity in children. These drugs, such as Phendimetrazine and Ritalin, are also sold in the illegal market and are used alone or in combination with other drugs, such as heroin.

Chronic amphetamine use, unlike chronic cocaine use, builds up tolerance so that eventually whole handfuls may be swallowed. Although excessive doses may cause psychoses, millions of Americans have taken amphetamines for a non-medical reason, such as staying awake to drive a truck or study for an exam, with few or no ill effects.

As for the effect of amphetamines on sex, they increase dopamine in the brain and dopamine is the neurotransmitter that interacts with serotonin to affect sexual-desire. The rush or high attained by snorting cocaine or mainlining "speed" has been compared to sexual stimulation or orgasm. When either is injected a man may have a spontaneous erection. When used before sexual intercourse, cocaine and amphetamines may facilitate a more intense experience and prolong the period until orgasm in both men and women. Women have reported that they experience an increase in the contractions of their vaginal muscles during orgasm.[1] These effects are dose related. Although the effects are generally correlated with the dose, larger doses being associated with more pronounced effects of sexual stimulation, increased energy, euphoria, and mental lucidity, large doses taken chronically, often result in impotence, insomnia, confusion, and anxiety, and eventually with amphetamines, little or no interest in sex.[2]

Downers: Barbiturates

As amphetamines are to cocaine, barbiturates are to alcohol. Barbs, like amphetamines, are legal drugs prescribed for a variety of problems. As amphetamines mimic the stimulant effect of cocaine, so barbs mimic the intoxication effects of alcohol. There is cross-tolerance between alcohol and barbiturates; if you can handle a lot of one, you can handle a lot of the other. Withdrawal symptoms are the same. Hangovers are the same. Behavior is the same. Thus we should not be surprised to find that barbs affect sexual function very much the way alcohol does. Like alcohol, a barb may increase desire but as Shakespeare noted in MacBeth when giving advice about "drink", "it provokes the desire but it takes away from the performance".

There are hundreds of barbiturates and their combinations. Their major differences are variations in the length of time before they take effect and the length of time their effects last. They are all central nervous system depressants.

The most commonly abused are Amytal (amobarbital), Nembutal (pentobarbital), and Seconal (secobarbital). Tuinal (a combination of amobarbital and secobarbital) is also abused. These pills begin acting 15-40 minutes after they are swallowed, and their effects last from 5-6 hours.

There are many street names for each of these barbs. They include bluebirds, dolls, downers, goofballs, sleepers, reds & blues, and tooties.

Because of their similarity to alcohol, barbiturates in small doses enhance libido by releasing inhibitions (called "disinhibition"). At doses large enough to induce heavy sedation and sleep, it would seem that barbiturate users wouldn't be interested in sex. But large doses of barbiturates produce a feeling of euphoria, called a downer high and it is this feeling that may sometimes be associated with sexual stimulation. In others, the same size dose produces only depression and apathy. Chronic use, like chronic alcohol use, often leads to impotence, loss of libido, and extending the time to climax.[3]

When young people in the drug subculture are asked about barbiturates, they say that barbs act like alcohol.[4,5] In small doses they decrease inhibitions and can produce euphoria, but they tend to make for sloppy sex, they delay ejaculations, and if the dosage is large enough, they cause impotence. The consensus is that, on average, barbs decrease sexual pleasure.

As one respondent said when responding to a questionnaire, "Depressants make sex rather undesirable and sloppy; sometimes it's just too much to do if you're downed out. On the occasions when sex has been completed, the act was very unsatisfactory (no real pleasure, sensations, or orgasm). The effect of alcohol is similar."[6]

In 1965 Quaalude (methaqualone) was the 6th most prescribed drug in the U.S. and was known in the sex and drug subculture as "the love drug". It was then considered to be a safer substitute for barbiturates. Eventually it was determined that "the love drug" was highly addictive, could cause convulsions, coma, and even death, and it was moved to Schedule I by the DEA in 1971.

Marijuana

Marijuana, including the cannabis plant and its cannabinoids, are listed in Schedule I. Pure tetrahydrocannabinol is also listed in Schedule III for limited uses, and sold as tablets under the brand name Marinol. Increasing numbers of states are permitting medical use of marijuana. In 2013, Colorado was the first state to control, tax, and sell marijuana in special stores for recreational use. However, such measures are state laws and have no effect on Federal law. Despite such changes in states, marijuana remains on Schedule I, effective across all U.S. states and territories.

The *United States Pharmacopeia,* which contains the most selective listing of the nation's drugs—no drug is admitted without the approval of a panel of independent expert physicians and pharmacologists—contains a monograph on "Extract of Hemp from 1850 to 1942." In the first half of this century, marijuana was prescribed for a wide range of medical conditions from gout to insanity, and especially for migraine headaches, and was contained in six widely prescribed products.

Many government commissions have carried out independent investigations of marijuana use. Their conclusions relative to why people use it are remarkably similar. Why do people smoke marijuana? Except for medical use, simple pleasure, similar to that claimed for the moderate use of alcohol or sex, is offered as the explanation for most marijuana use. "We do it for fun. Do not try to find a complicated explanation for it. We do it for pleasure."

"In the case of cannabis, the positive points which are claimed for it include the following: it is a relaxant; it is disinhibiting; . . . increases sensual awareness and appreciation; it is a shared pleasure . . ."

Next to alcohol, and often with it, marijuana is the most commonly used recreational drug in the United States and probably the world. The annual "Monitoring the Future" national high school survey reported in 2013 that over 36% of 12th graders had used marijuana at least once in the prior year. There are more than 40 street names for cannabis, the most common probably "grass", "pot", "herb", "weed", "Mary Jane". The moral outrage against marijuana in the early part of this century, which led to the ban of the drug, was not based on its use in medical practice, but because of a social revulsion against people using drugs recreationally. Alcohol was well entrenched in American society and survived prohibition as a legal psychotropic drug. Marijuana did not.[6]

More recently, and especially for medical use, marijuana is less likely to be smoked as a cigarette or via a bong but is vaporized and inhaled from a vaporizer thus avoiding carcinogenic substances such as smoke or tars. Demonstrations on where to obtain and use vaporizers and how to make them from items available at home are on *YouTube*.

Because sexual activity is also a widespread activity, it is certain that hundreds of thousands and probably millions of Americans have had sexual experiences while high on marijuana. But is marijuana an aphrodisiac? No. The mere fact that many people have sex after smoking marijuana does not make it one. Most grass smoking is not followed by sexual activity. The predominant pleasant effects of marijuana for most people is not sexual arousal but garrulousness, giddiness, warmth, mild euphoria, bouts of hilarity, heightened sense perceptions, enhanced visual and musical perceptions, time distortions, a feeling of good will, the "munchies", and what may be best described as a serene "spaciness."

Marijuana affects perceptions and feeling states during sexual activity. At the most it may predispose to sexual activity under certain conditions. It does not cause people to commit sexual acts or crimes. As one scientist commented, the problem is semantic. Does aphrodisiac mean to enhance manifest impulses, or does it mean to trigger preexisting impulses?[7] Marijuana fits the former but not the latter definition.

Most research on the effects of marijuana since the 1960s and 1970s have investigated harmful effects or medical uses and not users' reports of their feelings and experiences. However, in the late sixties, a State University of New York researcher asked two hundred marijuana users to fill in a questionnaire about how the drug affected them.[8] Almost 70 percent of the respondents said that marijuana enhanced their sexual response. Fewer, but more women than men, said that pot could excite their sexual interest. Half of the women and 39 percent of the men said that smoking marijuana could make them more interested in having sex, but this was only if the person they were smoking with was sexually desirable.

Both women and men said that marijuana had a pronounced effect on the quality of their physiological response during sexual intercourse. Women used terms like "intense," "ecstatic," "rhapsodic," some saying they experienced orgasm for the first time with marijuana. They said that marijuana made sex more beautiful, more spiritual, that there was greater sharing than without it.

Men said smoking marijuana extended the time of foreplay, that sex was more adventurous, that they could go on and on, lingering, enjoying every detail of the experience, that they had more control over ejaculation, and that when it happened it was a total, intense, orgasmic experience. One man said that sex lasted longer "by the clock." Regular marijuana users said they were more sexually affected than those who had only used it a few times.

In another survey investigating the sexual effects of marijuana, 750 questionnaires were given to students who were asked to pass them along until they fell into the hands of marijuana users who had smoked marijuana on 12 or more occasions.[9] Just over a fifth of the questionnaires were returned. Most of the persons wrote that marijuana very favorably enhanced their sexual pleasure, reporting in particular that their orgasm had developed new and more exciting qualities. They felt that the quality of their interpersonal relationships was improved, as well as physical sensations such as touch and taste. Commonly they reported that their sexual desire was increased in those situations where they would have been at least somewhat responsive, and that marijuana did not affect their sexual desire in those circumstances where it was inappropriate or if they did not like the persons who were potentially available. The survey concluded that, "For practically all experienced users, marijuana intoxication greatly intensifies the sensations experienced in sexual intercourse".

A rare survey not primarily of college students consisted of hippies who attended the free medical clinic in the Haight-Ashbury section of San Francisco. The director of the clinic asked known heavy drug users about the aphrodisiac properties of the various drugs they were using. Forty of the 50 men and women surveyed said that marijuana was the drug that most enhanced sexual pleasure. They said that sexual pleasure is only decreased in those few persons in whom marijuana causes anxiety or mild paranoia.[10]

The following are typical responses from 250 men and women who responded to ads in media such as *The Village Voice* asking them to respond to a survey on the effects of drugs, alcohol, and medicines on sexual function.[6] The youngest woman was 21 and the oldest was

46. Few women said that they smoked marijuana primarily for the way it affected them sexually. Typical responses were:

- "Social enjoyment—I like the reaction."
- "I enjoy smoking grass and do so most of the time."
- "Just to have a good time."
- "To relax."
- "Enjoyment, relaxation—it's really part of our life-style."
- "Relaxation, or as part of a social function."
- "Because it made things flow easier; for several years now I've had difficulty unwinding and relaxing to get into sex."
- "Just to get high."
- "Enjoy sensation. Never used for the purpose of improving sexual function."
- "To relax, be social; because I enjoy the way it makes me feel."

The ages of the men who filled in the questionnaire about their use of marijuana in association with sexual activity ranged from 22 to 56. All but one were experienced marijuana users, and most of them said that they had used the drug with alcohol. One of the men, aged 48, said he had tried smoking pot three times and the experience was so unpleasant he would never try it again. He said his heart pounded, and he became very frightened:

- "The room I was in was on the sixth floor. I felt that if I got out of my chair something terrible would happen—I might fall or jump out of the window. Then my wife came home and I wanted to make love because I had heard it was great with grass and I thought it might help. But she wouldn't because she was angry with me, and didn't understand why I was frightened, and I didn't want to tell her, so I got in bed and stayed there until the feelings went away. I don't think anyone should smoke grass by themselves for the first few times."

Like the women, the men said they did not use marijuana primarily for sex, but because they enjoyed getting high. Still, they recognized a contribution that marijuana could make to sexual pleasure:

- "I am extremely sensitive to THC [the active ingredient of marijuana] and it's not unusual for me to hallucinate after smoking one joint. The drug enables me to enter realms of my mind which are usually repressed by the demands of society. Not only are certain cerebral functions increased, but all sensations, thus sex is intensified. However, my primary reason for smoking is a fascination with my mind's ability to create, to analyze, and even to enter new dimensions."
- "Being high enhances any pleasurable sensations, making the sexual act just that much more enjoyable. Sex is immensely enjoyable anyway, but being high intensifies it."
- "I smoke marijuana regularly and often combine it with sex. It acts as an aphrodisiac for both of us."
- "To grasp for sensitivity and awareness not normally present."
- "Marijuana has an aphrodisiac effect, so sometimes I use it for this reason."
- "It is just different—a separate way."
- "The sexual aspects are just an added benefit to a pleasurable experience."
- "Sometimes I do [use it primarily for sex] because it's good for sex— but it's also good for other things."

The overall replies of men indicated they believe marijuana contributes to their sexual desire and arousal. Responses ranged from a simple "increased both," to the more descriptive:

- "Of all the psychotropic drugs I've used, marijuana has the greatest ability to stimulate my sexual desires, and especially after two or three successful attempts at coitus, it has the ability to renew my sexual interest. My touch becomes more sensitive, as though I had never touched the person before. My sexual desire increases and I have the opportunity to perform more coitus."

- "The effect was a strong feeling of closeness with the girl even though I hardly knew her. I felt like I loved her tremendously even though we were just having sex on a one night stand."
- "Usually any thought of sex while high would lead me on a pretty sustained track of desire and arousal."
- "My desire is vastly increased—especially when the person was in the room and had very few clothes on."
- "Although other drugs and alcohol increase my sexual drive too, marijuana seems to have the greatest effect on the height and renewal of desire and arousal."
- Orgasms are reported to increase in quality as well as number, several of the men attributing the difference between sex with marijuana and without it to changes in time perception:
- "Due to changes in temporal perspective, and the sensitizing nature of marijuana, orgasms are lengthy and very enjoyable."
- "The time it takes to have one depends more on the person I'm with. The quality is damn good."
- "The amount of time spent in foreplay and the quality of orgasm seemed to be increased. Perhaps this is due to altered time perception."
- "I tend to spend more time in foreplay—massaging, performing cunnilingus—when I am high. Such foreplay tends to enhance the quality of the total sexual experience. Climax is more intense after such foreplay."
- "There is more control and the orgasm lasts longer—it seems more dramatic and explosive and it feels better."
- "If I am very stoned, it will prolong my orgasm but not alter its intensity."
- "First orgasm achieved faster than when not high (2-3 minutes); second and third orgasms prolonged (10 minutes)."

When asked about the effect of marijuana on erections and ejaculations, the answers were somewhat more equivocal. Several men said it didn't have any effect at all, but one of these was the least enthusiastic about its effect on orgasm, saying only that "I guess it enhances its quality by opening your mind to the rush of emotions that you feel."

Others said erections were "stronger," "longer," "as many as orgasms," "increases size and hardness."

On balance, the consensus for the relationship of sex to grass is, "It's the one drug that's better than natural".[11] As one person put it, "Alcohol may make you think you want to more, but when you do it, you don't do as well. With grass it's just the opposite. It doesn't make you want to do it more, but when you do, it's better." As another put it, "Sexual orgasm has new qualities, pleasurable qualities. When making love I feel I'm in much closer mental contact with my partners; it's much more a union of souls as well as of bodies. I have no increase in sexual feeling unless it's a situation that I would normally be sexually aroused in, and then the sexual feelings are much stronger and more enjoyable. I feel as if I'm a better person to make love with when I'm stoned.[12]

In addition to time distortion, the principal effect of marijuana that contributes to increased sexual pleasure is probably that of touch, but the most important sex organ is the mind. If a drug like marijuana affects the mind, it will affect sexual function too. Whether the effects are perceived as good or bad depends on preexisting states, circumstances, and moral judgments.

The good news is that marijuana produces little physical dependence. That means that when habitual users stop, they have little physical symptoms or cravings such as those that develop with narcotic or alcohol addiction. Nor does tolerance develop. That means that people do not need larger and larger doses to feel an effect. If anything, the reverse seems to be true; habitual users need less to feel an effect. Marijuana produces no hangover or, indeed, any morning-after feelings at all. Certainly users may develop psychological dependence.

In addition to the anxiety state and feelings of fear and paranoia that marijuana produces in some people (bad trips!), other unpleasant side effects that have been associated with smoking marijuana are giddiness, rapid heartbeat, elevated blood pressure, loss of memory, delusions, nausea, throat and chest pains, dry mouth, and cold hands and feet.

In 1894, the Indian Hemp Drugs Commission Report concluded that, "the moderate use of these drugs is the rule", and that "the excessive use is comparatively exceptional. The moderate use practically produces no ill effects. In all but the most exceptional cases, the injury from habitual moderate use is not appreciable." No evidence has appeared since 1894 to challenge this statement.

Opioids

Opium itself and its constituents such as morphine and codeine and its derivatives such as heroin and synthetic substitutes such as methadone and Demerol (meperidine) or Dilaudid (hydromorphone), are all central nervous system depressants. They are downers. They are downers for sex. As a class, few drugs have more potential for making men impotent and women disinterested than do the opioids. Potential, however, is a critical word. Sexual functions may be damaged for those who are addicted and use opioids as a way of life— whose lives are run by their habit. For some of these persons, opioids can be a substitute for sex. For others, they are an escape from their sexual inadequacies.

Heroin is a Schedule I drug and thus is illegal in the U.S. Most of the other opioids are Schedule II unless combined with a NSAID or acetaminophen and are on Schedule III.

Opioid Generic Names	Opioid Brand Names
hydrocodone	Lortab, Norco, Vicodin
hydromorphone	Dilaudid, Paladone
meperidine	Demerol
methadone	Dolophine

Opioid Generic Names	Opioid Brand Names
morphine	Avinza, Kadian, MS Contin
oxycodone	OxyContin, Oxecta, Roxicodone
oxymorphone	Opana, Numorphan
tramadol	Ultram
Combination with hydrocodone: (with ibuprofen) Vicoprofen	
Combinations with oxycodone: (with acetaminophen) Endocet, Magnacet, Narvox, Percocet, Primlev, Roxicet, Tylex, Xolox; (with aspirin) Endodan, Percodan; (with ibuprofen) Combunox	

For some men, the dampening effect that opioids have on their sexual performance is enjoyed and welcomed; ejaculation can be blocked altogether or considerably delayed so that sexual intercourse can be prolonged almost indefinitely. This is one of the reasons that opium was very popular in India in the 1800s. About the time that opium was becoming a public health issue, morphine, especially injected morphine, was becoming the opiate of choice. Morphine is the chief active ingredient, and is about 10 percent of opium, so that it is about ten times stronger by weight than opium. Because it forms a soluble salt, it is injectable, unlike opium.

There is a strange history of opiates being used, or more appropriately misused, to treat addiction. Morphine was once prescribed to cure opium addiction, and heroin was subsequently prescribed to cure morphine addiction. Eventually the quality of cross-tolerance and cross-addiction among opioids became appreciated by the medical community, as it was early perceived by drug addicts. Next, along came methadone, another opioid, designed to substitute for heroin. Despite a prodigious search, the pharmaceutical industry has yet to produce a drug that has the analgesic, but not the addictive potential, properties of the opiates.

When morphine is given medically, it is often injected under the skin. By this route, the maximum pain-killing effect is reached in about half an hour, and the effect lasts from 4-6 hours. Actually opioids don't so much kill pain, in the sense of a local anesthetic, as they alter the perception of it. With opioids, people still know they are experiencing pain, but they feel detached from it. Anxiety drops away. Pain doesn't matter. Recreational opioid users or addicts prefer to mainline the drugs into a vein, because they get an immediate jolt, flash, or "rush" to the central nervous system. It is this rush that is often described in sexual terms and has caused the needle and the process of injection to take on sexual symbolism. The effects of narcotics shot into a vein have been described as "a total orgasm," or "an orgasm in the stomach."

Physical dependence means that the body's physiology has changed in response to a drug. As a diabetic needs insulin, and experiences physical symptoms when he does not get his injection, so an addict, if suddenly detached from his drug, experiences symptoms, such as restlessness, irritability, yawning, running nose and eyes, fever, chills and sweats, nausea, vomiting, diarrhea, insomnia, anorexia, and involuntary ejaculations.

Drug addicts are not great lovers. They may even have difficulty becoming parents. Of at least equal concern is the fact that an addicted pregnant woman produces a physically dependent infant.

Study after study have shown that long-term opioid addicts have substantial sex-related problems. Addicted men commonly experience erectile impotence, delayed ejaculation, failure to ejaculate, decreased nocturnal emission, and loss of sensitivity and sexual desire. Sperm motility is also suppressed.[13-16]

Women may experience difficulty attaining orgasm and have loss of desire.[17] Failure to menstruate is a common experience of female addicts.[18] However, they may actually become pregnant more often than non-addicted women because they become inattentive to the need for contraception.[14]

A little beyond the subject of this book, it has been speculated that the needle pain can be associated with masochistic symbolic orgasms. The injection substitutes for sex.[19] Thus, for those who have personality problems that mean they have difficulty forming relationships with others, "junk" can become a substitute for a sex partner. The junkie risks neither failure nor rejection. Junk is demanding but it always comes through.

Notably, all physical sex problems rapidly disappear when an addict goes drug-free. The problem is that sex is an inadequate substitute for drugs. Some addicts would rather have drugs than sex.

Perhaps no one said it better than Cocteau in 1930 in *Diary of a Cure*, ". . . there is no mistress more exacting than this drug which takes jealousy to the point of emasculating the addict. . . not only does it cause impotence, but what is more, it replaces these somewhat base obsessions by others which are somewhat lofty, very strange and unknown to a sexually normal organism".[20]

Inhalants

Although there are four categories of volatile inhalants, vaporizing liquids, sprays, gases, and nitrites, only the nitrites are related to sex. Amyl nitrite and other alkyl nitrites are used to treat heart diseases, and recreationally for their "rush" and prolongation of orgasm, particularly in males. They act directly on the central nervous system, brain, and spinal cord, relaxing blood vessels and causing blood pressure to drop. Amyl nitrite, the most popular, is used mainly as a sex enhancer.

The nitrites were prescription only status from 1937 to 1960 when they went OTC. There were more than 20 brands of amyl nitrite, butyl nitrite, and isobutyl nitrite sold OTC in the '60s but they were returned to prescription only status in 1969 in reaction to concerns about their recreational use. However, an exception was made for commercial use. Nitrites are in food preservatives, leather cleaner, room deodorizers, etc.. Their most common street name is "poppers" but they are also called "snappers".

Amyl nitrite relaxes the sphincter muscles of the anus and this is one of the reasons that it is a popular drug among male homosexuals. However, this is not the only reason that amyl nitrite is used in association with sexual function. It has a direct effect as well, producing a short but intense magnification of orgasm. Although some believe this is only because of the effect on the blood vessels of the sex organs, others say that the subjective experience of pleasure is too great for vasodilation to be the only reason, and that it results from a direct effect in the central nervous system as well.[21-23] Thus, amyl nitrite is not an aphrodisiac in the sense of increasing libido, but in the sense of modifying the sexual experience in pleasurable ways.

Butyl nitrite is not licensed or regulated by the FDA as a drug, but as a "room odorizer." However, unlike the floral or spice bouquets that one has a right to expect of a room odorizer, this one stinks of stale locker rooms and unwashed tennis shoes. As a room odorizer it is total humbug. As a recreational drug it has the same action as amyl nitrite, which smells a great deal better.

Butyl nitrite is not sold in neat little ampules, but in squat, wide-mouthed, screw-capped bottles that hold less than half an ounce. The label of at least one brand entices with its warning, "Danger. Excessive use may cause euphoria." The fumes may be sniffed directly from the bottle or through an inhaler that even has a lanyard attached, so it can be carried around the neck.

When people sniff these nitrites, they feel flushed, somewhat dizzy, and their hearts pound. In other words, they have the same kind of feelings they might have from frenzied dancing without nitrites. However, with the inhalant and dancing or sex at the same time, they are stimulated so they feel excited and passionate or wildly thrilled and ecstatic.

The most common side effect is a headache. Other unwanted effects–nausea, nasal irritation, cough, pounding pulse, dizziness, erectile impotence, and loss of emotional control–are relatively rare.

None of these effects lasts; only the headache may hang over to the next morning. Although blood pressure falls and heartbeat rate increases almost immediately upon inhalation, they usually both return to normal within two minutes.

According to one survey of 255 nitrite sniffers in the San Francisco Bay area, "The majority of volatile nitrite users have had at least one orgasm while under nitrite influence and report the experience to be intense, pleasurable and free of serious side-effects."[21]

A survey of men who had sex with men in the Baltimore-Washington, D.C., area reported that 69% had used an inhalant while having sex and 21% had done it in the prior year.[24]

Occasionally, men have a temporary loss of erection after inhaling the stuff, but that's not surprising considering that the volatile nitrites expand the blood vessels. After all, the penis is only held erect or tumescent because it is engorged with blood. If the passageways for blood expand and no more blood flows in to maintain the pressure, or if the expansion allows some of the blood to flow out, the pressure will drop and the penis will collapse.

Although not as visibly obvious, there's a parallel situation in women. Pooling of the blood in the genital area may be lessened so that the attainment of orgasm is inhibited. This suggests that women would not like the nitrites very much, but apparently some of them enjoy the overall body rush and heightened perceptions associated with inhalants.

Actually, it's hard to imagine women sniffing something that smells like decaying gym socks, as does butyl nitrite, and finding it romantic. That may be why there are more male than female nitrite sniffers, and why male users sniff more often than their female counterparts. Also, "poppers" and "room odorizers" are often sniffed just before the sexual climax. This method of operation seems O.K. for men who are relatively undistractible as they approach orgasm. Forget it for women though. If women are interrupted as they proceed toward orgasm, they tend to lose their edge and must almost start over to build toward climax. An interruption to take a whiff may be more of an interference than a welcomed adjunct.

Both amyl and butyl nitrite seem to be remarkably nontoxic. A clinical professor of psychiatry at the University of California reported the responses to a questionnaire sent to more than 3,000 emergency room physicians and more than 200 pathologists. The pathologists who responded said they had never seen a patient who died as a result of inhaling nitrites. Only thirteen of the emergency room physicians had seen any toxic reactions and these, headache, fainting, and low blood pressure, were short-lived.[22]

Anabolic Steroids

In common parlance these days you may hear something described as acting as though it's "on steroids." You probably won't want that something to be "sex on steroids" unless those steroids were prescribed to you for a medical condition.

There is no such thing as a strictly body building drug. Although anabolic steroids are derived from the naturally occurring male sex hormone, testosterone, men taking them may experience breast development, impotence, lower sperm count, acceleration of baldness, priapism (medical condition in which the erect penis does not return to its flaccid state), decrease in semen, and testicle atrophy (decrease in size). Women taking them become more like men as their voice deepens, their breasts shrink, they get more facial hair, they develop male pattern baldness, their menstrual cycle changes, and they have clitoral enlargement. Effectively, they are females turning male. Certainly, the adverse effects are related to dosage and how long they are taken. Although, most of the adverse effects are reversible once the user stops taking them, some are not.

Medical use includes delayed puberty, muscle loss from some

diseases, and male hormone problems, for example shrinking gonads. They may also be used for persons undergoing gender changes.

What are they? Anabolic steroids are technically called anabolic-androgenic steroids. Anabolic means "to build" and androgenic means "masculizing." Testosterone is the body's naturally occurring anabolic steroid. The rest are synthetic derivatives. There are also prohormones which metabolize into anabolic steroids after they are in the body. They are all classified as Schedule III drugs by the FDA.

It is estimated that 1% of the US population have misused anabolic steroids[25] and that 3% of American youth have used them.[26] They are taken, not only to build athletic abilities, but to improve appearance.[27]

As their use is banned in sports (doping) and their adverse side effects have become more recognized, many have been withdrawn from the legal market by pharmaceutical companies. An example is Winstrol (stanozolol) marketed by Winthrop whose official labeling listed 11 adverse reactions.[28]

Although there is a huge list of anabolic steroids that have been synthesized, some of which have been available legally in the past and may be available in the illegal market and in other countries. Wikipedia lists more than 50. The most common, and listed by the FDA, are Anadrol-50 (oxymetholone) a 50 mg tablet, Deca-Durabolin (nandrolone decanoate) in 50, 100, and 200 mg. tablets, Oxandrin (oxandrolone) in 2.5 and 10 mg tablets, and Winstrol (stanozolol) in 5 mg tablets and injections with 50, 75, and 100 mg per ml. Nandrox is an over-the-counter example of a prohormone that is said to metabolize into nandrolone in the body. There are also plants containing phytosteroids which may also metabolize into anabolic steroids. In addition, the FDA has approved an anabolic steroid for veterinary use, trenabolone, that is listed for human use along with many many other non-approved drugs in the Internet market.

Part Seven
Over-the-Counter Meds

16

Over-the-Counter and into the Bedroom

"The only thing we don't have is a good drug for premature-ejaculation...but I hear that it's coming quickly."

— Mel Brooks

There are two vastly different groups of OTC or Over the Counter drugs. None of these drugs requires a doctor's prescription and therefore may be sold directly to consumers at drugstores, supermarkets, convenience stores, on the web, through mail order and even door-to-door. One type of OTC drugs are those that have been on the market for many years (usually 20-25 or more) and usually began life as a prescription drug, but where experience over many years has shown that these medications are almost always used safely and so have been switched to OTC status.

The other "OTC" drugs are herbals, nutraceuticals and various supplements that make no specific curative claims, and therefore may also be sold freely at health food stores as well as elsewhere. There is much less known about this latter group, since they do not routinely undergo FDA-supervised formal clinical trials.

The typical OTC drugs are for common or non-serious conditions. Many of these medicines are for colds, cough, flu, pain, vitamin supplementation, allergies, and sleep aids. Others are for arthritis, overactive bladder, smoking cessation, or are minerals such as calcium for osteoporosis.

In addition to the oral OTC medications, there are numerous topical products such as creams and ointments for rashes, inflammatory conditions, callous and wart removal, hair removal, ear drops, eye drops and nasal sprays. The vast majority of topical medications are completely safe because they are applied at one spot and most of the medication remains in that general area. This is unlike an oral product such as a tablet that is digested and travels throughout the entire body.

The three major areas where OTCs might have an influence on sexual performance are with antihistamines, local anesthetics, and lubricants.

Antihistamines

Products containing antihistamines are commonly used to control allergic symptoms such as nasal congestion, watery eyes, and itching skin. The older antihistamines caused people to become sleepy and when people are sleepy, there is usually reduced interest in sex. Some of these drugs include Benadryl, (diphenhydramine), ChlorTrimeton, (chlorpheniramine maleate) and Tavist (clemastine). These antihistamines are available under hundreds of brand and generic names.

Local Anesthetics

The family of local anesthetics are the same drugs that your dentist uses to numb an area. Males sometimes use these ointments to desensitize the penis enabling them to take longer to reach orgasm. The anesthetic is normally applied before the condom is applied over it, protecting the partner from the medication, since the partner should not come into contact with the local anesthetic, as the partner does not need any parts to be numbed.

Some of the most common topical anesthetics are: lidocaine,

hemorrhoidal creams, benzocaine, tattoo numbing products, and prilocaine. These are available under a huge array of brand names.

Using too much local anesthetic cream or ointment can totally desensitize the penis and no arousal or ejaculation may occur.

Lubricants

You're getting old and your juices are drying or have dried up. WD-40 is not the answer. Instead you can visit your local pharmacy or super market and choose an over-the-counter lubricant from a large selection. They can be found in both the men's and women's areas, the men's usually side-by-side with the condoms. The women's usually with feminine hygiene products. Notably many of the same ones can be found in both these areas. Another source is the Internet.

The chain drug stores have their own labeled lubricants, usually cheaper versions of those with brand names. Frugal shoppers are wise to compare the ingredients listed on the labels and then compare the costs.

And remember the old standby, Vaseline? And the old saying, "Vaseline has a hundred and one uses. Everyone knows the one". Vaseline is petroleum jelly and it's labeled as a skin protectant. Petroleum jelly is also sold under many other brand names. Baby oil is another commonly used inexpensive lubricant for sex.

There are an astonishing number of lubricants now on the market. A visit to a chain pharmacy and super market revealed 17 different products, 5 with the chain pharmacy's own label. A visit to the Internet produced for females 27 more products under 10 more brand names. Adding in the ones listed for males and ones listed for both males and females, the total was 91 products. In addition to these, men may also use lubricated condoms.

On the Internet, one can choose products within categories. For women,

5 categories included: water based, silicone based, hybrid water/silicone based, added excitement, and anal lubes. The categories for men were the same as for women plus 4 more categories: oil based, delay lubes, flavored lubes, and hand gel/masturbation.

The issue relative to lubricants having different bases is their affect on condoms. Both oil-based and water-based lubricants may increase slippage of new and old condoms. Oil-based may increase breakage in either. Water-based lubricants don't affect the breakage rate of new condoms and decrease breakage of old ones. So if your condoms are new, it doesn't matter. If old, water-based is probably your better choice.

Let's look at some of the lubricants. Astroglide, one of the most popular, has an interesting history. It was developed by an engineer at Edwards Air Force Base in 1997 while he was working on NASA's space shuttle's cooling systems. It was not, as some rumors have it, developed for space sex.

What's in them? Astroglide has nine products, including gels, strawberry flavored, warming, and free of glycerin and parabens. Why free of glycerin and parabens? Because some men and women are allergic to them. Astroglide Liquid is water-based and includes glycerin, propylene glycol, polyquaternium15, methylparaben, and propylparaben. People with allergies, beware! Astroglide Natural, one of the 9 products, contains only plant-derived ingredients: xylitol, aloe vera, vitamins C and E, pectin (from fruit), and chamomile flower extracts. Another one made only of plant-derived ingredients is Aloe Cadabra, which is 95% aloe vera. Or there is Blossom Organics, which markets 5 products including gels, creams, oils. Their ingredients include sunflower seed oil, cinnamon oil, borage seed oil, menthol, vitamin B3, aloe leaf nectar, and various other substances such as hydroxymethylcellulose.

K-Y is another popular brand with 6 products under its label. They include K-Y Liquid, K-Y Jelly, K-Y Ultragel, K-Y Warming Liquid, K-Y

Warming Jelly, and K-Y Yours and Mine. K-Y Yours and Mine is packaged with two separate 1.5 fluid ounce containers, one for each. As promoted, when the ingredients come into contact, his "excites" and hers "delights".

What's in them?:

- K-Y Liquid or Jelly: propylene glycol, polyethyleneglycol, hydroxypropylene cellulose, tocopherol (Vitamin E).
- K-Y Jelly: glycerine, hydroxyethylcellulose, chlorhexidine gluconate, glucose lactone, methylparaben, and sodium hydroxide.
- Liquid Silk: water, propylene glycol, isopropyl palmitate, dimethicone, cellulose polymer, polysorbate 60, sorbitan stearate, cetearyl alcohol, glyceryl stearate nse, bnpd disodium edta, phenoxyethanol, methylparaben, butylparaben, ethylparaben, propylparaben, and bht
- Replens vaginal moisturer (with 14 applicators): water, glycerine, mineral oil, polycarbophil, carboner homopolymer Type B, palm oil glyceride, methyl paraben, sorbic acid, and sodium hydroxide.
- Trojan Lubricants Continuous Silkiness: proylene glycol, water, dimethicone/vinyl dimethicone crossover polymer, hydroxyethyl acrylate, socium acrylol taurate copolymer, methylparaben, and propylparaben
- Trojan Lubricants Arouses and Intensifies: dimethicone, dimethiconal, vanillyl butyl ether, menthol
- Trojan Lubricants Tingly Warmth: dimethicone, dimethiconol, hexyl nicotinate, and vanillyl butyl ether

And the rest? If you want to know the ingredients in any of the other lubricants, simply type their name into an Internet search engine such as Google, and you can probably find this information. As for choosing which one to buy, your best source for advice may be your physician.

Others

Aspirin, NSAIDs (non-steroidal anti-inflammatory drugs), multivitamins and most other OTC medications should be able to be used without worry of sexual performance problems. While OTCs have been proven safe, there is always a possibility that a person taking a prescription drug and an OTC or even two OTCs could be subject to a drug-drug interaction where two drugs used alone are fine, but when used together could be capable of causing a serious problem, even requiring hospitalization.

With the supplements and nutraceuticals, there is so much less information known to the pharmaceutical and medical communities that if a person begins taking a new drug in addition to the other medications they were previously using and some unusual reaction or pain or feeling begins, it is wise to consult one's pharmacist or physician. Tell your health professional what medications you have been taking and what product was just added, and then describe your reaction. The pharmacist, especially, can investigate this situation on your behalf. It is probably a good idea to skip a few doses of the new item until you get an all-clear message that the new medication is most likely not the culprit. If the problem resolves by itself simply by discontinuing the new medication, it is a pretty sure bet that the new drug was responsible.

Late night television, men's fitness and sports magazines and other media contain advertisements for mixtures of multiple vitamins, coenzymes and other compounds that claim to enhance men's performance regarding hardness and duration. Often there are 10 or more individual agents in such capsules, many of which have no clinical evidence of effectiveness. Caution is advised.

While nothing can be 100% true, speaking in generalities, consumers should feel confident that the drugs available OTC in the United States as laxatives, for diarrhea, for gastric reflux, for indigestion, headache, and most other OTC therapy areas should not be expected to have any positive or negative impact on one's sexual performance.

Part Eight
What You Can Do

17

Getting Help from Your Doctor or Pharmacist

"Tell me and I forget. Teach me and I remember. Involve me and I learn."

– Benjamin Franklin

No one is expected to know everything about all topics, and that includes physicians as well. The medical school curriculum is crowded and medical students have very limited opportunity to learn about some supplements, nutraceuticals and other home remedies. They gain additional knowledge and expertise during their residency training for several years in their chosen specialty area, and this is where the education of a physician gains a great deal of practical knowledge. When multiple patients complain about some symptoms and the physician discovers that the only common cause was some herbal product, he or she becomes suspicious and when that same symptom is presented by future patients, that doctor will surely ask whether the patient is using that herbal product. That is essentially how it works. Physicians become better and better as they gain practice experience.

Then there is the matter of who to trust. If you ask a roofing contractor if you need a new roof, there is often a high probability that you could predict the answer to your question. That situation is present if you ask a home insulation company if your house could use more insulation, or if you take advantage of a free check of your automatic transmission from an automatic transmission firm. It is likely that many persons bring in their cars for the "free" check-up will leave with some adjustments or repairs that are anything but free. The physician is the perfect person to ask questions about sexual performance medications or gadgets. Your physician has no vested interest in your spending of money and can be expected to provide you with an honest, unbiased, objective answer. If you ask whether a warming lubricant is effective, the physician will tell you what he or she knows, probably based upon what has been learned in practice over the years when other patients mentioned their happiness or displeasure with a product.

Of course, there will be instances when your physician has not heard about the product you are inquiring about, but they are often willing to point you in the direction of someone they know who might be able to answer your question or who can research the question. If you are going to ask about some capsules that promise to strengthen body parts, for example, it would be helpful for you to bring the bottle along with you at the time of your physician's appointment, or at a minimum, copy the list of ingredients from the label so the physician has the opportunity to evaluate each of the ingredients in the medicine before making any judgment.

You should not be embarrassed or ashamed as physicians deal with private, delicate, personal topics countless times every day. In fact, it is very likely that many others have asked the same question in the past, and an older physician may even have first-hand, personal experience in this matter. However, physicians cannot possibly keep up-to-date on every fad or rumor. In cases where one is considering using high doses of vitamins or other products already available as foods or as over-the-counter (OTC) products, the physician is likely to suggest that you investigate the idea carefully and to be on the lookout for any adverse events. That physician knows the power of placebos and realizes that something that cannot provide any pharmacologically based improvement can still help someone who believes in it. And who knows; perhaps the combination of ingredients does offer some benefit.

Another person where objective advice is possible is the community pharmacist. The pharmacist is a drug expert, and has reference resources nearby. The patient is pretty much assured of obtaining a truthful answer to inquiries. Pharmacists continue to be rated first or second in national polls about who the public trusts. A skeptic might ask whether the pharmacist profits by suggesting some product sold in the pharmacy, but that is only a remote possibility. The pharmacist is salaried and therefore cannot possibly gain by the sale of a $10.00 or $20.00 item. As with the case of physicians, pharmacists improve their ability to assist patrons from the feedback they receive from patients who often report back that a product helped or did not help. Of course, the privacy available at the physician's office is not possible at the pharmacy counter, but that negative point has to be balanced against the advantages of convenience with no required appointment, 24/7 availability of the pharmacist and no fee for an office visit.

In any case, one should not be afraid or be too timid to ask a healthcare professional for help. The only bad question is the question that is not asked.

18

Good Medical Information Sources

"Knowledge is of two kinds. We know a subject ourselves, or we know where we can find information upon it".

– Samuel Johnson

People don't ask for a number of reasons, including concern about fees, lack of pharmacist or physician access, timidity, fear of divulging personal or sensitive information, privacy, embarrassment or the unwillingness to discuss personal matters with others, there are, fortunately, other sources for help. Twenty years ago, this chapter would have advised you to go to the library or local bookseller. But today, there is a wide array of sources available, which do not require leaving the comfort and relative privacy of one's home. Many worldwide web sites do not require registering or providing any personal or identifiable information, giving the person with a question a high degree of anonymity. A private web communication should ideally be anonymous and confidential.

Today, using the web for health information often yields too much information and the sources need to be vetted. A manufacturer of male enhancement products can be expected to maintain a website under "male enhancement products," that appears to be neutral, non-commercial, and academic or scholarly. But the consumer must exercise extreme caution. The first job then is to obtain a list of possible sites and the second job is to cull it so that only the most reliable and informative sites remain in your final list. This second chore may be most easily accomplished by asking yourself what the website sponsor has to gain from the information provided. So, government and international agencies may offer more complete or reliable information than, for example, the producer of a libido stimulating capsule.

What follows is a sampling of some sites reviewed by the editors of this book in 2014. At that time, the site's information was checked and what follows was considered accurate. However, things change over time and you, the reader, are urged to use your judgment when inquiring about a sexual performance question.

Search Engines

At the moment, there are three main search engines which a typical computer user has access to. They are: Google.com, Ask.com, Bing.com

The lion's share of the search engine business goes to Google.com, but it is worthwhile to check a second or third site if you are still having difficulty in finding a credible source for the information you are seeking, since it is not uncommon to find that one or another of those principal search engines just might have a source not available through the others. The old adage that you have to ask the right question if you want the right answer holds true for online searches as well. Let's say that you want to know about warming lubricants. You will need to check out that topic "warming lubricants," but it would be useful to also look into "personal lubricants," "sexual lubricants," etc. Just think of all of the terms that come to mind, and you can ask a specific question, such as: "What do you look for in selecting a personal lubricant," or " What are the advantages of warming lubricants?"

If you find scientific articles from professional societies or from academic sources, they usually explore very specific questions and you should read the 1-2 paragraph abstract to determine whether it might be fruitful to read the complete 6-15 page full article. In most cases, you will not need to go beyond reading only the abstract.

Specific Sites: (Presented in no specific order)

Erectile dysfunction - Viagra.com has a great deal of information, as is the case for its competitor products, Cialis and Levitra, to name a few, from their respective websites.

www.healthline.com is a comprehensive website that provides information and guidance for a wide array of medical problems, and it is highly regarded for its accuracy.

www.wickipedia.org is a popular website that covers many of the most common sexual performance issues for men and women. It also provides the original references it uses, so that the serious person can follow-up further in greater depth.

www.webmd.com is another popular site that covers a diverse spectrum of sexual and medical issues among a very thorough list of non-sexual health topics. It is easy to use and it is understandable by non healthcare professionals.

www.amazon.com for two areas. Amazon carries an incredible assortment of books on sexual and medications topics, and it also sells performance enhancing products for women and men. Its descriptions of those products are quite thorough and objective.

The website of the American Sexual Health Association is worth a visit for general background information and for referrals to other reference sources. It is rich with professionally approved information and it offers an opportunity to learn the conventional wisdom on various topics.

Perhaps, one of the most valuable resources on the web is the site of the Mayo Clinic. At the Diseases and Conditions section of its website, one may learn a great deal of up-to-date information and suggestions about any topic one might imagine.

A book, the Merck Manual, describes the diagnosis, treatment and prognosis for just about any medical condition known to man or woman. It helps physicians decide between two conditions with similar symptoms. Some advanced level laypersons use it to research problems within their own families.

www.healthfinder.gov is a splendid website that helps ordinary people determine how to navigate the complex and often confusing world of health websites and information sources. It is maintained by the US federal government and is nearly always useful; sometimes in unexpected ways.

Another very helpful website is found at www.health.nih.gov which has in-depth information about many important medical conditions. It does not include every sexual health issue, but it is worth checking if one is having difficulty finding answers elsewhere.

One of the most well regarded sites is the one produced by the University of California San Francisco (UCSF) Medical School – www.ucsfhealth.org>Patient Education. It is accurate, up-to-date, and quite easy to use and understand.

A very down-to-earth site is www.familydoctor.org which colleagues report is very user-friendly and well written.

www.fda.gov/drugs/resources is a real treasure of drug information. Various parts of the FDA website tell us if a drug has been approved and if so, when and for what conditions. It contains sections on fraud, OTC drugs and problems.

There is a website maintained by the National Institute of Aging that describes some problems and medical issues faced by senior citizens. It contains a great deal of background and introductory information but is quite limited in the area of drugs for sexual performance enhancement.

The Medical Library Association has a splendid website that helps one find reliable sources for health questions.

The European Medicines Agency (EMA), the European counterpart of the US Food and Drug Administration (FDA) has a superb website understandable by anyone. It has much information about drugs that have been approved and in Europe, that might not have been approved for sale in the USA yet. This is a useful website to contact when one is offered a product that someone tells you is not available in the USA.

The US Federal Trade Commission (FTC) runs a website that has a section "Health Information for Older People." It is worth visiting if the situation calls for it. It provides fine advice and guidance to help visitors discern what is useful and objective in other websites.

The Better Business Bureau (BBB) maintains a list of complaints about products and services. These lists are available and can be valuable in helping one determine whether or not to buy some advertised item.

One of the most robust websites is that one from the World Health Organization (WHO), a United Nations agency. Unfortunately, it takes quite a while to navigate it to find specific answers and to get through so much information. One of its more valuable pieces is the list of Essential Drugs.

The United Nations maintains a list of drugs banned anywhere in the world. It can be found on the UN website and one can verify if any ingredients in a product has been banned in any other country.

www.CHPA.org is the website of the over-the-counter drug manufacturers association. It lists reports and studies and press releases about non-prescription drugs.

www.intelihealth.com would be a worthwhile site where some sexual effects of drugs might be found. In addition, it contains a world of other valuable information on numerous other health topics. It accesses the American Hospital Pharmacy Formulary.

www.drugs@FDA.gov provides official labeling of FDA approved drugs in the USA, which sometimes includes information about their effects on sex.

If it becomes necessary to check original scientific journal articles from the clinical literature, a marvelous site is the collection of the US National Library of Medicine. It is accessed through PUBMED at www.ncbi.nlm.nih.gov/pubmed. You will have to experiment with different keywords unless you know the name of an author of an article, but it is quick and easy to use and perhaps the most comprehensive health information site anywhere. Also, you may obtain an abstract or the complete paper by email almost immediately.

There are countless other sites and hundreds of textbooks that have not been mentioned. The reason for that is not any lack of confidence in many of the other sources, but rather a practical effort not to overwhelm the reader. The sites listed above are among the ones that this book's editors consult more often than others.

Appendices

Appendix A: Most Frequently Prescribed Drugs and Sex Effects

* Capitalized drugs are brand names; others are generics. If your drug has no page number, the authors found no reports in the scientific literature of that drug having sex effects.

Most Frequently Prescribed Drugs and Sex Effects			
Drug Name	Page	Drug Name	Page
Abilify	90, 93	Amytal	104
Acebutol	67	Anadrol	120
Aciphex	*	Androderm	35
Activase	*	Androgel	35
Actos	*	Apri	53
Adderall	102	Aranesp	90, 93
Adderall XR	102	aripiprazole	90-93
Advair Disc	*	Asacol	*
Advair HFA	*	atenolol	67, 72
Advicor	77	Ativan	88
Aggrenox	*	atorvastatin	75
Alesse	53	Atripla	*
Alimta	*	Aurorix	84
Allopurinol	*	Avantyl	*
alprazolam	87	Avapro	73
Altocor	75	Avastin	*
amiloride	67	Aviane	53
amineptine	85	Avinza	114
amitriptyline	84	Avodart	*
amlodipine	72	Avonex	*
amnestrogen	45	Axiomin	82
amobarbital	104	azithromycin	*
amoxicillin	*	Benicar	*
amphetamine	100-103	Benzapril	67

| Most Frequently Prescribed Drugs and Sex Effects ||||
Drug Name	Page	Drug Name	Page
Benzedrine	102	clonidine	73
Betaseron	*	clozapine	90,92
betaxolol	67	Clozaril	90
Bezafibrate	*	Colcrys	*
Bezalip	76	Combivent	*
bisoprolol	67,73	Compactin	75
Brevicon	53	Complera	*
Brintellix	82	Covaryx	45
budesonide	*	Crestor	75
Bumex	67	cyclobenzaprine	*
bupropion	83	Cymbalta	*
Buspar	88	cyproterone	58
buspirone	43,87,88	Dalmane	87
Byetta	*	dapoxetine 80	80
Caduet	*	Deca-Durabolin	120
captopril	67	Demulen 53	53
carteolol	67	Demerol	113
Carvedilol	67,72	Depo-Provera	62
Celebrex	*	desipramine	*
Cenestin	*	Desogen	53
cephalexin	*	Desyrel	*
Chantix	*	DetrolLA	*
chlorazepate	87	dexedrine	102
chlordiazepoxide	87,89	Dexilant	*
chlorpromazine	90,92	dextroamphetamine	102
Cialis	28,31-34,37,73,77,78	Dextrostat	102
cimetidine	*	diazepam	87
Ciprodex	*	Didrex	102
ciprofibrate	*	digoxin	*
Citalopram	80	Dilaudid	113
Claravis	*	Diovan	68
clomipramine	85	Diuril	67
clonazepam	87	Dolophine	113

Most Frequently Prescribed Drugs and Sex Effects			
Drug Name	**Page**	**Drug Name**	**Page**
Doral	88	Fetzima	82
doxepine	83	Flovent HFA	*
dyrenium	72	fluconazole	*
Edromax	81	fluphenazine	90
Effexor	82	flurazepam	87
Effient	*	fluoxetine 80	80
Eldepryl	83-94	fluvastatin	75
Eloxatin	*	fluvoxamine 80	80
enalapril	67, 72	FocalinXR	*
Enbrel	*	Forteo	*
Enjuvia	46	Fosinopril 67	67
Enoxaparin	*	furosemide	72
Epipen	*	gabapentin	*
Epogen	*	Gammagard	*
Epzicom	*	GamunexC	*
Equanil	88	Gardasil	*
Erbitux	*	gemfibrozil	*
escitalopram	*	Genora 53	53
Essian	45	Geodon	91, 94
Estrace	46	Gilenya	*
Estratest	45	Gleevec	*
Estrostep	53	Halcion	88
Estrostep Fe	53	Haldol	91, 92
Eurodin	87	haloperidol	91, 92
Evex	46	Herceptin	*
Evista	*	Humalog	*
Exelon	*	hydromorphone	113
Fazaclo	90	Hygroton	67
felodipine	73	Hypnovel	88
Femogen	46	ibuprofen	*
Femtest	46	imipramine	*
fenofibrate	*	Incivek	*
fenofibric acid	*	indapamide	73

Most Frequently Prescribed Drugs and Sex Effects			
Drug Name	Page	Drug Name	Page
Invega Sustenna	91, 93	losartan	73
Isentress	*	lovastatin	75
isocarboxazid	*	Lovaza	*
Ixel	*	Lovenox	*
Janumet	*	Low-Ogestrel 53	53
Januvia	*	loxapine	91
Jenest-28	53	Loxitane	91
Juvisync	76	Lozol	67
Ketipinor	91, 93	Lucentis	*
Klonopin	87	Lunesta	*
Korlym	61	Lybrel	53
Lantus	*	Lyrica	*
Lasix	67, 72	marijuana	100, 102, 105-113
Lescol	75	Marplan	84
Levemir	*	Maxalt	*
Levitra	28, 31-34, 37, 42	meloxicam	*
Levlen	53	Menest	46
Levora	53	Menogen	46
levothyroxine	*	meperidine	113
Lexapro	80, 83	meprobamate	45, 88
Lexiscan	*	metazolone	67
Librium	87, 89	metformin	*
Lidoderm	*	methadone	113
Lipex	75	methaqualone	105
Lipitor	75, 77, 78	methyldopa	73
lisinopril	67, 72	methylprednisolone	*
Livalo	75	metopolol	72, 73
Lo/Ovra	53	Mevacor	75
Loestrin	53	mevastatin	75
Loestrin Fe	53	Microgestin	53
Lopid	76	Microgestin Fe	53
lorazepam	87	Micronor	54
Lortab	113	Midamar	67

Most Frequently Prescribed Drugs and Sex Effects				
Drug Name	**Page**	**Drug Name**	**Page**
midazolam	88	Norpace	96
mifeprex	61	Norpramin	*
Miltown	88	Nortrel	53
Mircette	53	nortriptyline	85
Mirena	62	Nor-QD	54
Modalim	76	Norvir	*
Modecate	90	Novolog	*
Modicon	53	Numorphan	114
moexipril	67	NuvaRing	62
morphine	113, 114	Ogestrel	53
Motrin	*	olanzapine	92, 93
MS Contin	114	omeprazole	*
Namenda	*	Onglyza	*
Naproxen	*	Opana	114
Nardil	83, 84	opipramol	85
Nasonex	*	Orencia	*
Navane	91	Ortho Tri-Cyclen	53
nebivolol	72, 73	Ortho-Cept	53
Necon	53	Ortho-Cyclen	53
nefazodone	*	Ortho-Novum	53
Nembutal	104	Ortho-Novum	53
Neulasta	*	Ortho-Novum	53
Neupogen	*	Osphena	44, 45
Nexium	*	Ovcon	53
Nexplanon	62	Ovral	53
Niaspan	*	Ovrette	54
nitrazepam	88	Oxandrin	120
Nizoral	96	oxazepam	88
Norco	*	Oxecta	114
Nordette	53	oxycodone	114
Norinyl	*	Oxycontin	114
Normarex	82	oxymorphone	114
Normison	88	Paladone	113

| Most Frequently Prescribed Drugs and Sex Effects ||||
Drug Name	Page	Drug Name	Page
Pantoprazole	*	ProairHFA	
ParaGard	62	ProCentra	102
Parnate	*	prochlorperazine	91
paroxetine	80	ProComp	91
Paxil	80	Procrit	*
Pegasys Pk	*	promethazine	*
Pentazine	91	ProSom	87
pentobarbital	104	protriptyline	85
Peragal	91	Provigil	
Percocet	114	Prozac	80
Percodan	114	Psigodal	*
perindopril	67	quazepam	88
Pernazinum	91	quetiapine	91-93
perphenazine	91	quinapril	67
phendimetrazine	103	Ramipril	67
phenelzine	*	ranitidine	*
Phenergan	91	Rebif	*
Pirazidol	*	Reclast	*
pirlindol	*	Remeron	81
pitavastatin	75	Remicade	*
Plan B 61	61	Restasis	*
Plavix	*	Restoril	88
PotassiumCl	*	Revela	*
Pradaxa	*	Revlimid	*
Pramolan	*	Reyataz	*
Pravachol	75	Risperdal	91-93
pravastatin	75	risperidone	91-93
prazepam	88	Ritalin	103
prednisone	*	Rituxan	*
Premarin	44-46	rosuvastatin	75
Prevnar	*	Roxicodone	114
Prezista	*	Seasonale	53
Pristiq	82	Seasonique	53

Most Frequently Prescribed Drugs and Sex Effects			
Drug Name	**Page**	**Drug Name**	**Page**
secobarbital	104	Syntest	
Seconal	104	Tagamet	96
selegiline	*	testosterone	4-6, 10, 15, 27, 30, 32-35, 40-42, 59, 77, 92, 96, 119
Selektine	75	Thorazine	90, 92
Semap	91	Tianeptine	85
Sensipar	*	tiotixene	91
Serax	88	Tofranil	84
Serdolect	91, 94	Tolvan	81
Serlect	91, 94	Torvast	75
Seroquel	91, 94	tramadol	114
sertindole	91, 92, 94	trandolapril	67
Sertraline	*	Tranxene	87
Servector	*	tranylcypromine	*
Serzone	82	trazodone	82
Simcor	76	Treanda	*
Simponi	*	triamterine	*
simvastatin	75, 77, 78	triazolam	88
Singulair	*	TriCor	76
Solodyn	*	trifluoperazine	*
Sordinol	90	Trilafon	91
Spiriva	*	Tri-Levlen	91
spironalactone	67	Trilipix	76
Stablon	*	trimipramine	85
Stelara	*	Tri-Norinyl	*
Stelazine	91	Triphasil	53?
Stendra	28, 33, 34, 37	Trivora	53?
Strattera	81	Truvada	53?
Suboxone	*	Tuinal	104
Surmontil	*	Ultram	114
Sutent	*	Valdoxan	83
Symbicort	*	Valium	87
Synagis	*	Varuvax	*

Most Frequently Prescribed Drugs and Sex Effects			
Drug Name	**Page**	**Drug Name**	**Page**
Velcade	*	Zoloft	32, 80
venlaxfaxine	*	Zolpidem	*
VentolinHFA	*	Zometa	*
Versed	88	Zostavax	*
Verstram	87	Zyban	83
Vesicare	29, 30	Zyprexa	91, 93
Viagra	27-37, 39, 42, 93	Zytiga	*
Vicodin	*	Zyvox	*
Vidaza	*		
Vimpat	*		
Viread	*		
Vitamin D	*		
Vivactil	*		
Vivalam	81		
Vytorin	76		
Vyvanse	102		
Yasmin	*		
Yas Zovia	*		
warfarin	*		
Welchol	*		
Wellbutrin	*		
Xanax	87, 89		
Xeloda	*		
Xgeva	*		
Xifaxan	*		
Xolair	*		
Yervoy	*		
Zeldox	94		
Zetia	*		
ziprasidone	91, 94		
Zocor	75, 77		

Appendix B: References

Chapter 1

1. Okabe M. The cell biology of mammalian fertilization. *Development* 140:4471-9, 2013.
2. Yiee JH, Baskin LS. Penile embryology and anatomy. *Sci World J* 10:1174-9, 2010.
3. Hsieh CH, Liu SP, Hsu GL, et al. Advances in understanding of mammalian penile evolution, human penile anatomy and human erection physiology: clinical implications for physicians and surgeons. *Med Sci Monitor: Intl Med J Exp Clin Res* 18:RA118-25, 2012.
4. Awad A, Alsaid B, Bessede T, Droupy S, Benoit G. Evolution in the concept of erection anatomy. *Surg Radiol Anat* 33:301-12, 2011.
5. Mawhinney M, Mariotti A. Physiology, pathology and pharmacology of the male reproductive system. *Periodontology 2000* 61:232-51, 2013.
6. Setchell BP. The Parkes Lecture. Heat and the testis. *J Repro Fertility* 114:179-94, 1998.
7. Griswold MD, Oatley JM. Concise review: Defining characteristics of mammalian spermatogenic stem cells. *Stem Cells* 31:8-11, 2013.
8. Kim B, Kawashima A, Ryu JA, Takahashi N, Hartman RP, King BF, Jr. Imaging of the seminal vesicle and vas deferens. *Radiographics* 29:1105-21, 2009.
9. Gonzales GF. Function of seminal vesicles and their role on male fertility. *Asian J Androl* 3:251-8, 2001.
10. Sullivan R, Saez F. Epididymosomes, prostasomes, and liposomes: their roles in mammalian male reproductive physiology. *Reproduction* 146:R21-35 2013.
11. Corona G, Jannini EA, Vignozzi L, Rastrelli G, Maggi M. The hormonal control of ejaculation. *Nature Rev Urol* 9:508-19, 2012.
12. McArdle CA. Gonadotropin-releasing hormone receptor signaling: biased and unbiased. *Mini Rev Med Chem* 12:841-50, 2012.
13. Menon KM, Menon B. Structure, function and regulation of gonadotropin receptors - a perspective. *Molec Cell Endocrinol* 356:88-97, 2012.

14. Sriraman V, Rao AJ. FSH, the neglected sibling: evidence for its role in regulation of spermatogenesis and Leydig cell function. *Indian J Exper Biol* 43:993-1000, 2005.
15. Kuhn S, Gallinat J. A quantitative meta-analysis on cue-induced male sexual arousal. *J Sex Med* 8:2269-75, 2011.
16. Althof SE, Perelman MA, Rosen RC. The Subjective Sexual Arousal Scale for Men (SSASM): preliminary development and psychometric validation of a multidimensional measure of subjective male sexual arousal. *J Sex Med* 8:2255-68, 2011.
17. Koukounas E, Over R. Habituation of male sexual arousal: effects of attentional focus. *Biol Psych* 58:49-64, 2001.
18. Sachs BD. Contextual approaches to the physiology and classification of erectile function, erectile dysfunction, and sexual arousal. *Neurosci Biobehav Rev* 24:541-60, 2000.
19. Amann RP. Considerations in evaluating human spermatogenesis on the basis of total sperm per ejaculate. *J Androl* 30:626-41 2009.
20. Ferretti A, Caulo M, Del Gratta C, et al. Dynamics of male sexual arousal: distinct components of brain activation revealed by fMRI. *NeuroImage* 26:1086-96, 2005.
21. Redoute J, Stoleru S, Gregoire MC, et al. Brain processing of visual sexual stimuli in human males. *Human Brain Map* 11:162-77, 2000.
22. Rupp HA, Wallen K. Sex differences in response to visual stimuli. A review. *Arch Sex Behav* 37:206-18, 2008.
23. Cera N, Di Pierro ED, Sepede G, et al. The role of left superior parietal lobe in male sexual behavior: dynamics of distinct components revealed by FMRI. *J Sex Med* 9:1602-12, 2012.

Chapter 2
1. Puppo V. Anatomy and physiology of the clitoris, vestibular bulbs, and labia minora with a review of the female orgasm and the prevention of female sexual dysfunction. *Clin Anat* 26:134-52, 2013.
2. Puppo V. Embryology and anatomy of the vulva: the female orgasm and women's sexual health. *Eur J Obstet Gynecol Repro Biol* 154:3-8, 2011.
3. Giuliano F, Rampin O, Allard J. Neurophysiology and pharmacology of female genital sexual response. *J Sex Marital Ther* 28 Suppl 1:101-21 2002.
4. Jannini EA, Rubio-Casillas A, Whipple B, Buisson O, Komisaruk BR, Brody S. Female orgasm(s): one, two, several. *J Sex Med* 9:956-65, 2012.
5. O'Connell HE, Sanjeevan KV, Hutson JM. Anatomy of the clitoris. *J Urol* 174:1189-95, 2005.
6. Battaglia C, Nappi RE, Mancini F, et al. Menstrual cycle-related morphometric and vascular modifications of the clitoris. *J Sex Med* 5:2853-61, 2008.
7. Colvin CW, Abdullatif H. Anatomy of female puberty: The clinical relevance of developmental changes in the reproductive system. *Clinical anatomy* 26:115-129, 2013Strohbehn K. Normal pelvic floor anatomy. *Obstet Gynecol Clin North Amer* 25:683-705, 1998.
8. Strohbehn K. Normal pelvic floor anatomy. *Obstet Gynecol Clin North Amer* 25:683-705, 1998.

9. O'Connell HE, Eizenberg N, Rahman M, Cleeve J. The anatomy of the distal vagina: towards unity. *J Sex Med* 5:1883-91 2008.
10. Farage M, Maibach H. Lifetime changes in the vulva and vagina. *Arch Gynecol Obstet* 273:195-202, 2006.
11. Ashton-Miller JA, Delancey JO. On the biomechanics of vaginal birth and common sequelae. *Ann Rev Biomed Eng* 11:163-76 2009.
12. Parikh M, Rasmussen M, Brubaker L, et al. Three dimensional virtual reality model of the normal female pelvic floor. *Ann Biomed Eng* 32:292-6, 2004.
13. Ludmir J, Sehdev HM. Anatomy and physiology of the uterine cervix. *Clin Obstet Gynecol* 43:433-9, 2000.
14. Cicinelli E, Einer-Jensen N, Galantino P, Alfonso R, Nicoletti R. The vascular cast of the human uterus: from anatomy to physiology. *Ann NY Acad Sci* 1034:19-26, 2004.
15. Lyons RA, Saridogan E, Djahanbakhch O. The reproductive significance of human Fallopian tube cilia. *Human Repro Update* 12:363-72 2006.
16. Oktem O, Oktay K. The ovary: anatomy and function throughout human life. *Ann NY Acad Sci* 1127:1-9, 2008.
17. Edgardh K, Ormstad K. The adolescent hymen. *J Repro Med* 47:710-4, 2002.
18. Goodyear-Smith FA, Laidlaw TM. What is an 'intact' hymen? A critique of the literature. *Med Sci Law* 38:289-300, 1998.
19. Kilchevsky A, Vardi Y, Lowenstein L, Gruenwald I. Is the female G-spot truly a distinct anatomic entity? *J Sex Med* 9:719-26, 2012.
20. Flamini MA, Barbeito CG, Gimeno EJ, Portiansky EL. Morphological characterization of the female prostate (Skene's gland or paraurethral gland) of Lagostomus maximus maximus. *Ann Anat* 184:341-5, 2002.

Chapter 3
1. Bachtel MK. Do hookups hurt? Exploring college students' experiences and perceptions. *J Midwifery Womens Health* 58:41-8, 2013.
2. Nelson AL, Purdon C. Non-erotic thoughts, attentional focus, and sexual problems in a community sample. *Arch Sex Behav* 40:395-406, 2011.
3. Rowland DL, Georgoff VL, Burnett AL. Psychoaffective differences between sexually functional and dysfunctional men in response to a sexual experience. *J Sex Med* 8:132-9 2011.
4. Park SY, Bae DS, Nam JH, et al. Quality of life and sexual problems in disease-free survivors of cervical cancer compared with the general population. *Cancer* 110:2716-25 2007.
5. Abdel-Nasser AM, Ali EI. Determinants of sexual disability and dissatisfaction in female patients with rheumatoid arthritis. *Clin Rheumatol* 25:822-30 2006.
6. Chervenak JL. Reproductive aging, sexuality and symptoms. *Seminars Repro Med* 28:380-7 2010.
7. Taylor MJ, Rudkin L, Bullemor-Day P, Lubin J, Chukwujekwu C, Hawton K. Strategies for managing sexual dysfunction induced by antidepressant medicine. *The Cochrane database of systematic reviews* 5:CD003382 2013.
8. Schmidt HM, Hagen M, Kriston L, Soares-Weiser K, Maayan N, Berner MM.

Management of sexual dysfunction due to antipsychotic drug therapy. *The Cochrane database of systematic reviews* 11:CD003546 2012.
9. Fooladi E, Bell RJ, Davis SR. Management strategies in SSRI-associated sexual dysfunction in women at midlife. *Climacteric* 15:306-16 2012.
10. Nunes LV, Moreira HC, Razzouk D, Nunes SO, Mari Jde J. Strategies for the treatment of antipsychotic-induced sexual dysfunction and/or hyperprolactinemia among patients of the schizophrenia spectrum: a review. *J Sex Marital Ther* 38:281-301 2012.
11. Gutierrez MA, Mushtaq R, Stimmel G. Sexual dysfunction in women with epilepsy: role of antiepileptic drugs and psychotropic medicines. *Intl Rev Neurobiol* 83:157-67 2008.
12. Labbate LA. Psychotropics and sexual dysfunction: the evidence and treatments. *Adv Psychosom Med* 29:107-30 2008.
13. Nurnberg HG. An evidence-based review updating the various treatment and management approaches to serotonin reuptake inhibitor-associated sexual dysfunction. *Drugs of Today* 44:147-68 2008.
14. Balami J, Robertson D. Parkinson's disease and sexuality. *British journal of hospital medicine* 68:644-647 2007.
15. Higgins A. Impact of psychotropic medicine on sexuality: literature review. British journal of nursing 16:545-550 2007.
16. Thomas DR. medicines and sexual function. *Clin Geriatric Med* 19:553-62 2003.
17. Stewart ST, Cutler DM, Rosen AB. US trends in quality-adjusted life expectancy from 1987 to 2008: combining national surveys to more broadly track the health of the nation. *Amer J Public Health* 103:e78-87 2013.
18. Schmidt B, Ribnicky DM, Poulev A, Logendra S, Cefalu WT, Raskin I. A natural history of botanical therapeutics. *Metabol Clin Exper* 57:S3-9 2008.
19. Halberstein RA. Medicinal plants: historical and cross-cultural usage patterns. *Ann Epidemiol* 15:686-99 2005.
20. Raskin I, Ribnicky DM, Komarnytsky S, et al. Plants and human health in the twenty-first century. *Trends Biotech* 20:522-31 2002.
21. Drew AK, Myers SP. Safety issues in herbal medicine: implications for the health professions. *Med J Australia* 166:538-41 1997.
22. Gurwitz JH, Field TS, Harrold LR, et al. Incidence and preventability of adverse drug events among older persons in the ambulatory setting. *J Amer Med Assoc* 289:1107-16 2003.
23. Wilkinson GR. Drug metabolism and variability among patients in drug response. *New Eng J Med* 352:2211-21 2005.
24. Yan Z, Caldwell GW. The current status of time dependent CYP inhibition assay and in silico drug-drug interaction predictions. *Curr Topics Med Chem* 12:1291-7 2012.
25. Almond LM, Yang J, Jamei M, Tucker GT, Rostami-Hodjegan A. Towards a quantitative framework for the prediction of DDIs arising from cytochrome P450 induction. *Curr Drug Metab* 10:420-32 2009.
26. Hellum BH, Hu Z, Nilsen OG. The induction of CYP1A2, CYP2D6 and CYP3A4 by six trade herbal products in cultured primary human hepatocytes. *Basic Clin Pharmacol Toxicol* 100:23-30 2007.

27. Gray S, West LM. Herbal medicines–a cautionary tale. *New Zealand Dental J* 108:68-72 2012.
28. Abad MJ, Bedoya LM, Bermejo P. An update on drug interactions with the herbal medicine Ginkgo biloba. *Curr Drug Metabo* 11:171-81 2010.
29. Pergolizzi JV, Jr., Labhsetwar SA, Puenpatom RA, Joo S, Ben-Joseph R, Summers KH. Exposure to potential CYP450 pharmacokinetic drug-drug interactions among osteoarthritis patients: incremental risk of multiple prescriptions. *Pain Practice* 11:325-36 2011.

Chapter 5

1. Meuleman E, Cuzin B, Opsomer RJ, Hartmann U, Bailey MJ, Maytom MC, Smith MD, Osterloh IH. A dose-escalation study to assess the effectiveness and safety of sildenafil citrate in men with erectile dysfunction. *BJU Internat* 87:75-81, 2001.
2. Benchekroun A, Faik M, Benjelloun S, Bennani S E, Mirini M, Smires A. A baseline-controlled open-label flexible dose-escalation study to assess the safety and efficacy of sildenafil citrate (Viagra®) in patients with erectile dysfunction. *Int J Impot Res Suppl* 15(1):S19, 2003.
3. Buvat J, Hatzichristou D, Maggi M, Farmer I, Martinez-Jabaloyas J, Miller PJ, Schnetzler G. Efficacy tolerability and satisfaction with sildenafil citrate 100-mg titration compared with continued 50-mg dose treatment in men with erectile dysfunction. *BJU Internat* 102:1645-50, 2008.
4. Benard F, Carrier S. Lee JC, Talwar V, Defoy I. Men with mild erectile dysfunction benefit from sildenafil treatment. *J Sex Med* 7:3725-35, 2010.
5. Park HJ, Park NC, Shim HB, Park J.K, Lee SW, Park K, Kim SW, Moon KH, Lee DH, Yoon SJ. And open-label musltcenter flexible dose study to evaluate the efficacy and safety of sildenafil citrate (Viagra) in Korean men with erectile dysfunction and arterial hypertension who are taking antihypertensive agents. *J Sex Med* 5:2405-13, 2008.
6. DeYoung L, Chung E, Kovac JR, Romano W, Brock G., Daily use of sildenafil improves endothelial function in men with type 2 diabetes. *J Androl* 33(2):176-80, 2012.
7. Safarinejad M., Taghiva A, Shekarchi B, Safarinelad S.. Safety and efficacy of sildenafil citrate in the treatment of Parkinson-emergent erectile dysfunction: a double-blind placebo-controlled randomized study. *Int J Impot Res* 5:325-35, 2010.
8. Spitzer M, Basaria S, Travison TG, Davda MN, Paley A, Cohen B, Mazer N, Knapp PE, Hanka S, Lakshman K., UlloorJ, Zhang A, Orwoll K, Eder R, Collins L, Mohammed N, Rosen R.C, DeRogatis L, BhasinS. Effect of testosterone replacement on response to sildenafil citrate in men with erectile dysfunction: a parallel randomized trial. *Ann Intern Med* 20:681-91, 2012.
9. Li WQ, Qureshi AA, Robinson KC, Han J. Sildenafil use and increased risk of incident melanoma in US men: a prospective cohort study. *JAMA Intern Med* 174(6):964-70, 2014.
10. Sanford M. Vardenafil orodispersible tablet. *Drugs* 71(1):87-8, 2012.

11. Dubruyne FM, Gittelman M, Sperling H, Borner M, Beneke M. Time to onset of action of vardenafil: a retrospective analysis of the pivotal trials for the orodispersible and film-coated tablet formulations. *J Sex Med* 8:2912-23, 2011.
12. Mirone, Vincenzo, Palmieri, Allesandro, Cucinotta, Domenico, Parazzine, Fabio, Morelli, Montorsi, Francesco, Fexible-dose vardenafil in a community-based population of men affected by erectile dysfunction: A 12-Week Open-Label Multicenter Trial. *J Sex Med* 2:842-7, 2005.
13. Martin-Morales A, Graziottin A, Jaoude GB, Debruyne F, Buvat J, Benekd M, Neuser D. Improvement in sexual quality of life of the female partner following vardenafil treatment of men with erectile dysfunction: a randomized, double-blind, placebo-controlled study. *J Sex Med* 8:2831-40, 2011.
14. Sperling H, Debruyne F, Boermans A, Beneke M, Ubrich E, Ewald S. The POTENT I randomized trial: efficacy and safety of an orodispersible vardenafil formulation for the treatment of erectile dysfunction. *J Sex Med* 7(4 Pt 1): 1497-507, 2010.
15. Kendirci M, Bivalacqua TJ, Hellstrom WJ. Vardenafil: a novel type 5 phosphodiasterase inhibitor for the treatment of erectile dysfunction. *Expert Opin Pharmacother* 5:923-32, 2004.
16. Crowe SM, Streetman DS. Vardenafil treatment for erectile dysfunction. *Ann Pharmacother* 38(1): 77-85, 2004.
17. Morales AM, Mirone V, Dean J, Costa P. Vardenafil for the treatment of erectile dysfunction: an overview of the clinical evidence. *Clin Interv Aging* 4:463-72, 2008.
18. Kamenov ZA. Comparison of the first intake of vardenafil and tadalafil in patients with diabetic neuropathy and diabetic erectile dysfunction. *J Sex Med* 8:851-64, 2011.
19. Javaroni V, Queiroz MM, Burla A, Oigman W, Neves MF. Response to on-demand vardenafil was improved by its daily usage in hypertensive men. *Urology* 80:858-64, 2012.
20. Aversa A, Francomano D, Bruzziches R, Natali M, Guerra A, Latini M, Donni LM, Lenzi A. A pilot study to evaluate the effects of vardenafil on sexual distress in men with obesity. *Int J Impot Res* 24:122-5, 2012.
21. Mathers MJ, Klotz T, Roth S, Lummen G, Sommer F. Safety and efficacy of vardenafil versus sertraline in the treatment of premature ejaculation: a randomized, prospective and crossover study. *Andrologia* 41(3):169-75, 2009.
22. Gokce A, Demirtas A, Halis F, Ekmekciogfu O. In vitro measurement of ejaculation latency time (ELT) and the effects of vardenafil on ELT on lifelong premature ejaculators: placebo-controlled, double-blind, cross-over laboratory setting. *Int Urol Naphrol* 42:881-7, 2010.
23. Aliaev IuG, Vinarov AZ, Akhvlediani ND Choice of treatment of erectile dysfunction associated with hypogonadism. *Urologia* 4:37-8, 40-2, 1020.
24. Porst H, Hell-Momeni K, Buttner H. Chronic PDE-5 inhibition in patients with erectile dysfunction - a treatment approach using tadalafil once-daily. *Expert Opin Pharmacother* 13:1481-94, 2012.
25. Li JP, Li F, Guo WB, Zhou QZ, Mao XM, Tan WL, Zheng SB. Efficacy of low-dose tadalafil on ED assessed by Self-Esteem and Relationship Questionnaire. *Zhonghue Nan Kie Xue* 16:1147-9 2010.

26. Xu WD, Liu ZY, Ye HM, Lu X, Su CL, Ji JT, Piao SG, Sheng X. Efficacy and safety of lont-term small-dose tadalafil in the treatment of erectile dysfunction. *Zhonghue Nan Kie Xue* 17:531-4, 2011.
27. Tang, YX, Zhour HB, Peng SL, Jian XZ, He LY, Li DJ. Effects of tadalafil on erectile dystunction: on-demand versus once-daily dosing. *Zhonghue Nan Kie Xue* 18:472-4, 2012.
28. Wang XK, Luo L, Wang S, Li J, Li WX. Tadalafil improves total testosterone, IIEF score and SEP in old and middle-aged males with late-onset hypogonadism. *Zhonghue Nan Kie Xue* 18:475-7, 2012.
29. Gokce MI, Gulpinar O, Ozturk E, Gulec S, Yaman O. Effect of atorvastatin on erectile functions in comparison with regular tadalafil use. A prospective single-blind study. *Int Urol Nephrol* 44:683-7, 2012.
30. Yu H, Wu H, Rao D. Analysis of the therapeutic effect of tadalafil on male ED after transurethral resection of prostate. *Int J Impot Res* 24:147-9, 2012.
31. Oudiz, RJ, Brundage, BH, Galie N, Ghofrani HA, Simonneau G, Botros FT, Chan J, Beardsworth A, Barst RJ, PHIRST Study Group. Tadalafil for the treatment of pulmonary arterial hypertension: a double-blind 52-week uncontrolled extension study. *J Am Coll Cardiol* 21:768-74, 2012.
32. Morales AM, Casillas M, Turbi C. Patients' preference in the treatment of erectile dysfunction: a critical review of the literature. *Int J Impot Res* 23:970-85, 2011.
33. Alwaal A, Al-Mannie R, Carrier S. Future prospects in the treatment of erectile dysfunction: focus on avanafil. *Drug Des Develop Ther* 5:435-43, 2011.
34. Limin M, Johnsen N, Hellstrom WJ. Avanafil, a new rapid-onset phosphodiesterase 5 inhibitor for the treatment of erectile dysfunction. *Expert Opin Invest Drugs* 19:1427-37, 2010.
35. Goldstein I, Jones LA, Belkof LH, Karlin GS, Bowden CH, Peterson CA, Trask BA, Day WW. Aanafil for the treatment of erectile dysfunction: a multicenter, randomized, double-blind study in men with diabetes mellitus. *Mayo Clin Proc* 87:843-52, 2012.
36. Hellstrom WJ, Freier MT, Serefoglu EC, Lewis RW, DiDonato K, Peterson CA. A phase II, single-blind, randomized, crossover, evaluation of the safety and efficacy of avanafil using visual stimulation in patients with mild to moderate erectile dysfunction. *BJU Int* 111:137-47, 2013,
37. Rizio N, Tran C, Sorenson M. Efficacy and satisfaction rates of oral PDE5is in the treatment of erectile dysfunction secondary to spinal cord injury: a review of literature. *J Spinal Cord Med* 35(4):219-28, 2012.
38. Lombardi G, Nelli F, Celso M, Mencarini M, Del Popolo G. Treating erectile dysfunction and central neurological diseases with oral phosphodiesterase type 5 inhibitors. Review of the literature. *J Sex Med* 9:970-85, 2012.
39. Puma JL. Don't ask your doctor about "Low T". *New York Times* Op-Ed, pg A19, 2 Feb 2014.
40. Corona G, Rastrelli G, Forti G, Maggi M. Update in testosterone therapy for men. *J Sex Med* 8:639-54, 2011.
41. Chen J, Wollman Y, Chernichovsky T, Iaina A, Sofer M, Matzkin H. Effect of oral administration of high-dose nitric oxide donor L-arginine in men with organic

erectile dysfunction: results of a double-blind, placebo-controlled study. *BJU Int* 83(3):269-73, 1999.
42. Ernst E, Posadzki P, Lee MS. Complementary and alternative medicine (CAM) for sexual dysfunction and erectile dysfunction in older men and women: an overview of systematic reviews. *Maturitas* 70:37-41, 2011.
43. Jackson G, Arver S, Banks I, Stecher VJ. Counterfeit phosphodiesterase type 5 inhibitors pose significant safety risks. *Int J Clin Pract* 64:497-504, 2010.

Chapter 6

1. Simon JA. Low sexual desire - is it all in her head? Pathophysiology, diagnosis, and treatment of hypoactive sexual desire disorder. *Postgrad Med* 122:128-36, 2010.
2. Gerritsen J, van der Made F, Bloemers J, van Ham D, Kleiverda G, Everaerd W, Olivier B, Levin R, Tuiten A. The clitoral photoplethysmograph: a new way of assessing genital arousal in women. *J Sex Med* 6:1678-87, 2009.
3. Congalen HM, O'Connor EJ, McCae MP, Conaglen JV. An investigation of sexual dysfunction in female partners of men with erectile dysfunction: how interviews expand on questionnaire responses. *Int J Impot Res* 22:355-62, 1010.
4. Schmidt HM, Hagen M, Kriston L, Soares-Weiser K, Maayan N, Berner MM. Management of sexual-dysfunction due to antipsychotic drug therapy. *Cochrane Data Base Syst Rev* 11:CD003546, 2012.
5. Fabre LF, Smith LC, DeRogatis LR. Gepirone-ER treatment of low sexual desire associated with depression in women as measured by the DeRogatis Inventory of Sexual Function (DISF) fantasy/cognition (desire) domain- a post hoc analysis. *J Sex Med* 8:2569-81, 2011.
6. Bancroft J, Doll HA, Greco T, Tanner A. Does oral contraceptive-induced reduction in free testosterone adversely affect the sexuality or mood of women? *Psychoneuroendocrinology* 32:246-55, 2007.
7. White WB, Grady D, Giudice LC, Berry SM, Zborowski J, Snabes MC. A cardiovascular safety study of LibiGel (testosterone gel) in postmenopausal women with elevated cardiovascular risk and hypoactive sexual desire disorder. *Am Heart J* 163:27-32, 2012.
8. van der Made F, Bloemers J, Yassem WE, Kleiverda G, Everaerd W, van Ham D, Olivier B, Koppeschaar H, Tuiten A. The influence of testosterone combined with a PDE5-inhibitor on cognitive, affective, and physiological sexual functioning in women suffering from sexual-dysfunction. *J Sex Med* 6:777-90, 2009.
9. Taylor MJ, Rudkin L, Bullemor-Day P, Lubin J, Chakwujekwu C, Hawton K. Strategies for managing sexual-dysfunction induced by antidepressant medication. *Cochrane Data Base Syst Rev* May 11, 2013.
10. Hobbs K, Handler L. Clinical inquiry: which treatments hellp women with reduced libido? *J Fam Pract* 62:102-3, 2013.
11. Jayne C, Simon JA, Kimura T, Lesko LM. Open-label extension study of filbanserin in women with hypoactive sexual desire disorder. *J Sex Med* 9:3180-8, 2012.
12. Katz M, Derogatis LR, Ackerman R, Hedges P, Lesko L, Garcia M Jr., Sand M. *J Sex Med* May 14, 2013 (doi:10.1111/jsm.12189 Epub).

13. Derogatis LR, Komer L, Katz M, Moreau M, Kimura T, Garcia M Jr., Wunderlich G, Pyke R. Treatment of hypoactive sexual desire disorder in premenopausal women: efficacy of filbanserin in the VIOLET study. *J Sex Med* 9:1074-85, 2012.
14. FDA News Release. FDA approves Osphena for postmeno-pausal women experiencing pain during sex. U.S. Food and Drug Administration. 02-26-2013.
15. Kokot-Kierepa M, Bartuzi A, Kulik-Rechberger B, Rechburger T. Local estrogen therapy-clinical implications-2012 update. *Ginekol Pol* 62:102-3, 2013.

Chapter 7

1. Bush PJ: The placebo effect, JAPhA NS14:671-74, 1974. Reprinted in *Nursing Digest* 4:12-15, 1976.
2. Bush PJ: Case 16: *Placebos*. In Smith MC, Wertheimer AI: *A Casebook in Social and Behavioral Pharmacy*. Cincinnati, OH: Harvey Whitney Books, 1987.
3. Moerman DE, Jonas WB, Bush PJ et al.: Placebo effects and research in alternative and conventional medicine. *Chinese J Integ West Med* 2(2):141-8, 1996.

Chapter 8

1. Herzberg BN, Draper KC, Johnson AL, *et al*. Oral contraceptives depression, and libido. *Brit Med J* 3:495-500, 1971.
2. Dennerstein L, Burrows G. Oral contraception and sexuality. *Med J Australia* 1:796-8, 1976.
3. O'Dwyer WF. (Letter) Oral contraceptives, depression, and libido. *Brit Med J* 3:702, 1971.
4. Davis AR, Castano PM. Oral contraceptives and libido in women. *Ann Rev Sex Res* 15:297-320, 2004.
5. Robinson SA, Dowell M, Pedulla D, McCauley L. Do the emotional side-effects of hormonal contraceptives come from pharmacologic or psychological mechanisms? *Med Hypoth* 63:268-73, 2004.
6. Pastor Z, Holla K, Chmel R. The influence of combined oral contraceptives on female sexual desire: a systematic review. *Eur J Contracept Reprod Health Care* 18:27-43, 2013.
7. Burrows LJ, Basha M, Goldstein AT. The effects of hormonal contraceptives and women's sexuality: a review. *J Sex Med* 9:2213-23, 2012.
8. Battaglia C, Battaglia B, Mancini F, Busacchi P, Paganotto MC, Morotti E, Venturoli S. Sexual behavior and oral contraceptives: a pilot study. *J Sex Med* 9:550-7, 2012.
9. Higgins JA, Hoffman S, Graham CA, Sanders SA. Relationships between condoms, hormonal methods, and sexual pleasure and satisfaction: an exploratory analysis from the Women's Well-Being and Sexuality Study. *Sex Health* 5:321-30, 2008.
10. Adams DB, Gold AR, Burt AD. Rise in female-initiated sexual activity at ovulation and its suppression by oral contraceptives. *New Engl J Med* 299: 1145-50, 1978.
11. Enzlin P, Weyers S, Janssens D, Poppe W, Felen C, Pazmany E, Elaut E, Amy

JJ. Sexual functioning in women usuig levonorgestrel-releasing intrauterine systems as compared to copper uterine devices. *J Sex Med* 9:11065-73, 2012.

Chapter 9

1. Manolis A, Doumas M. Sexual dysfunction: the 'prima ballerina' of hypertension-related quality of life complications. *J Hypertens* 26(11):2074-84, 2008.
2. Scranton RE, Goldstein I, Stecher VJ. Erectile dysfunction diagnosis and treatment as a means to improve medication adherence and optimize comorbidity management. *J Sex Med* 10(2):551-61, 2013.
3. Manolis A, Doumas M. Antihypertensive treatment and sexual-dysfunction. *Curr Hypertens Rep* 14(4):285-92, 2012.
4. Bulpitt C J, Dollery CT. Side effects of hypotensive agents evaluated by a self-administered questionnaire. *Brit Med J* 3:485-90, 1973.
5. Mustafaev II, Nurmamedova GS. Effect of monotherapy with nebivolol, bisoprolol, carvedilol on the state of vegetative nervous system and sexual function in men with arterial hypertension. *Kardiologiia* 53(2):48-54, 2013.
6. Chen U, Cui A, Lin J, Xu Z, Zhu W, Shi L, Yang R, Wang R, Dai Y. Losartin improves erectile dysfunction in diabetic patients: a clinical trial. *Int J Impot Res* 24(6):217-20, 2012.
7. Vertkin AL, Vilkovyskii FA, Skotnikov AS, Zviagintseva EI, Skotnikova EV. Medical and social implications of sexual dysfunction and safety of antihypertensive therapy in hypertensive patients. *Kardiologiia* 51(10):46-52, 2011.
8. Yang LO, Yu J, Ma RX, Liu PJ, Guo XY, Li, XL, Chang P, Hu H, Zhao F, Bai F. Effect if different combined antihypertensive regimen on the erectile function in male hypertensive patients. *Zhonghua Xin Xue Guan Bing Za Zhi* 39(7):636-41, 2011.
9. Xu D, Yu J, Liu PJ, Guo XY, Hu H, Chang P, Li XL, Zhao F, Chen XH, Shen XP, Zhang Y, Bai F. Effect between felodipine plus irbesartan and felodipine plus metoprolol regimen on the sexual function in young and middle-aged women with hypertension. *Zhonghua Xin Xue Guan Bing Za Zhi* 38(8):728-33, 2010.
10. Saigitov RT, Glezer MG. Effect of arterial hypertension on sexual health of men and their qualaity of life. Results of BOLERO study. *Kardiologiia* 49(9):44-50, 2009.
11. Mills L C. Drug-induced impotence. *Amer Fam Prac* 12:104-6, 1975.
12. Laver M C. Sexual behaviour patterns in male hypertension. *Aust NZ J Med* 4:29-31, 1974.
13. Bauer G E, Hull RD, Stokes GS, Raftos J. The reversibility of side effects of guanethidine therapy. *Med J Aust* 1:930-33, 1973.
14. Newman RJ, Salerno HR. (Letter) Sexual dysfunction due to methyldopa. *Br Med. J* 4:106, 1974 Horwitz D, Pettinger WA, Orvis H. Effects of methyldopa in fifty hypertensive patients. *Clin Pharmaco. Therap* 8:224-34, 1967.
15. Karavitakis M, Komninos C, Theodorakis PN, Politis V, Lefakis G, Mitsios K, Koritsiadis S, Doumanis G. Evaluation of sexual function in hypertensive men receiving treatment: a review of current guideline recommendations. *J Sex Med* 8(9):2405-14, 2011.

Chapter 10

1. Golomb BA, Evans MA. Statin adverse effects : a review of the literature and evidence for a mitochondrial mechanism. *Am J Cardiovasc Drugs* 8:373-418, 2008.
2. Rizvi K, Hampson JP, Harvey JN. Do lipid-lowering drugs cause erectile dysfunction? A systematic review. *Family Pract* 19:95-98, 2002.
3. Neel AB. 7 meds that can wreck your sex life. www.AARP.org/health,4/25/12.
4. Solomon H, Samarasinghe YP, Feher MD, Man J, Rivas-Toro H, Lumb PJ, Wierzbicki AS, Jackson G. Erectile dystunction and statin treatment in high cardiovascular risk patients. *Intl J Clin Prac* 60:141-5, 2006
5. Trivedi D, Kirby M, Wellsted DM, Ali S, Hackett G, O'Connor B, van Os S. Can simvastatin improve erectile function and health-related quality of life in men aged ≥ 40 years with erectile dystunctin? Results of the Erectile Dysfunction and Statins Trial. *BJU Int* 111:324-33, 2013.
6. Gokce MI, Gulpmar O, Ozturk E, Gulec S, Yaman O. Effect of atorvastatin on erectile functions in comparison with regular tadalafil use. A prospective single-blind study. *Int Urol Nephrol* 44:683-7, 2012.
7. Hong SK, Han BK, Jeong SJ, Byun SS, Lee SE. Effect of statins therapy on early return of potency after nerve sparing radical retropubic prostatectomy. *J Urol* 178:613-6, 2007.
8. Herrmann HC, Levine LA, Macaluso J Jr, Walsh M, Bradbury D, Schwartz S, Mohler ER 3rd, Kimmel SE. Can atorvastatin improve the response to sildenafil in men with erectile dysfunction not initially responsive to sildenafil? Hypothesis and pilot trial results. *J Sex Med* 3:303-8, 2006.
9. Dadkhah F, Safarinejad MR, Asgari MA, Hosseini SY, Lashay A, Amini E. Atorvastatim improves the response to sildenafil in hypercholesterolemic men with erectile dysfunction not initially responsive to sildenafil. *Int J Impot Res* 22:51-60, 2010.
10. Mastalir ER, Carvalhal GF, Portal VI. The effect of simvastatin in penile erection: a randomized, double-blind, placebo-controlled clinical trial. *Int J Impot Res* 23:242-8, 2011.

Chapter 11

1. Galecki P, Florkowski A, Depko A, Wozniak A, Talarowska M. Characteristic and treatment of sexual dysfunctions in depression (part I). *Pol Merkur Lekarski.* 31(183):193-6, 2011.
2. Clayton AH, Montejo AL. Major depressive disorder, antidepressants, and sexual dysfunction. *J Clin Psychiatry* 67 Suppl 6:33-7, 2006.
3. Abdel-Hamid IA. Pharmacologic treatment of rapid ejaculation: levels of evidence-based review. *Curr Clin Pharmacol* 1:243-54, 2006.
4. Payne RE, Sadovsky R. Identifying and treating premature ejaculation: importance of the sexual history. *Cleve Clin J Med* 74 Suppl 3:47-53, 2007.
5. Targonski A, Prajsner A. Treatment of premature ejaculation. *Wiad Lek* 65:44-7, 2012.

6. Porst H. An overview of pharmacotherapy in premature ejaculation. *J Sex Med* 4 Suppl 4:335-41, 2011.
7. Watanabe N, Omori IM, Nakagawa A, Cipriani A, Barbui C, Churchill R, Furukawa TA. Cochrane Database Syst Rev 12:CD006528, 2011. Mirtazapine versus other antidepressive agents for depression.
8. Gurkan L, Oommen M, Hellstom WJ. Premature ejaculation: current and future treatments. *Asian J Androl* 10:102-9, 2008.
9. Avarez E, Vinas F. Mitazapine in combination. *Actas Esp Psiquiatr* 38(2):121-8, 2010.
10. Fagiolini A, Comandini A, Catena Dell'Ossa, Kaspar S. Rediscovering trazodone for the treatment of major depressive disorder. *CNS Drugs* 26(12):1033-49, 2012.
11. Baldo P, Doree C, Molin P, McFerran D, Cecco S. Antidepressants for patients with tinnitus. *Cochrane Database Syst Rev* 12:CD003853, 2012.
12. Dhillon S, Yang LP, Curran MP. Bupropion: a review of its use in the management of major depressive disorder. *Drugs* 68(5):653-89, 2008.
13. Rapaport MH, Thase ME. Translating the evidence on atypical depression into clinical practice. *J Clin Psychiatry* 68(4):e11, 2007.
14. Segraves RT. Pharmacological agents causing sexual dysfunction. *Sex Marital Therap* 3:157-76, 1977.
15. Gwin RD. O'Haram G L. Drug-induced changes in sexuality. *Apothecary* (Jan/Feb):11-60, 1978.
16. Simpson G M., Blair J H, Amuso D. Effect of anti-depressants on genito-urinary function. *Dis Nerv Syst* 26:787-89, 1965.
17. Wyatt RJ, Fram DH, Buchbinderm R et al. Treatment of intractable narcolepsy with a monoamine-oxidase inhibitor. *New Engl J Med.* 285:987-91, 1971.
18. Ruskin DB, Goldner RD. Treatment of depressions in private practice with imipramine. *Dis Nerv Syst* 20:391-99, 1959.
19. Shochet BR. Medical aspects of sexual dysfunction. *Drug Therapy* (Jun):37, 1976.
20. Greenberg, HR. Erectile impotence during the course of Tofranil therapy. *Amer J Psychiatr* 121:1021, 1965.
21. Leucht C, Huhn M, Leucht S. Amitriptyline versus placebo for major depressive disorder. *Cochrane Database Syst Rev* 2;12:CD009138, 2012.
22. Rowland DL, Tai WL, Brummett K, Slob AK Predicting responsiveness to the treatment of rapid ejaculation with 25 mg. clomipramine as needed. *Int J Impot Res* 16(4):354-7, 2004.
23. Shafey H, Atteya A, el-Magd SA, Hassanein A, Fathy A. Tianiptine can be effective in men with depression and erectile dysfunction. *J Sex Med* 3(5):910-7, 2006
24. Clayton AH, Montejo AL. Major depresssive disorder, antidepressants, and sexual dysfuncton. *J Clin Psychiatry* 67 Suppl 6:33-7, 2006.
25. Bodnar S, Catterill TB. Amitriptyline in emotional states associated with the climacteric. *Psychosomatics* 13:117-19, 1972.
26. Kerr MM. Amitriptyline in emotional states at the menopause. *NZ Med* 72:243-45, 1970.

Chapter 12

1. Page C, Michael C, Sutter M, Walker M, Hoffman BB. *Integrated Pharmacology* (2nd ed.). C.V. Mosby, 2002.
2. Olkkola KT, Ahonen J. Midazolam and other benzodiazepines. *Handbook of Experimental Pharmacology* 182:182, 2008.
3. Dikeos DG, Theleritis CG, Soldatos CR. "Benzodiazepines: effects on sleep". In Pandi-Perumal SR, Verster JC, Monti JM, Lader M, Langer SZ (eds.). *Sleep Disorders: Diagnosis and Therapeutics*. Informa Healthcare. pp. 220–2, 2008.
4. Ezine Articles.com/2272033.
5. Greenberg HR. Inhibition of ejaculation by chlorpromazine. *Nerv Ment Dis* 152:364-6, 1971.
6. Hughes J M. Failure to ejaculate with chlordiazepoxide. *Amer J Psychiatr* 121:610-11, 1964.

Chapter 13

1. Licitsyna OG, Ansseau M, Gernay P, Pitchot W, Bertrand J. Sexual dysfunction induced by antidepressants and antipsychotics. *Ter Arkh* 84(10):103-8, 2012.
2. Schmidt HM, Hagen M, Kriston L, Soares-Weiser K, Maayan N, Berner MM. Management of sexual dysfunction due to antipsychotic drug therapy. *Cochrane Database Syst Rev* Nov 14;11:CD003546, 2012.
3. Nunes LV, Moreira HC, Razzouk D, Nunes SO, Mari Jde J. Strategies for the treatment of antipsychotic-induced sexual dysfunction and/or hyperprolactinemia among patients of the schizophrenia spectrum. *J Sex Marital Ther* 38(3):281-301, 2012.
4. Inder WJ, Castle D. Antipsychotic-induced hyperprolactemia. *Aust NZ J Psychiatry.* 45(10):830-7, 2011.
5. Komossa K, Rummel-Kluge C, Schwarz S, Schmid F, Hunger H, Kissling W, Leucht S. Risperidone versus other atypical antipsychotics for schizophrenia. *Cochrane Database Syst Rev.* Jan 19;(1):CD006626, 2011.
6. Serretti A, Chniesa A. A meta-analysis of sexual dysfunction in psychiatric patients taking antipsychotics. *Int Clin Psychopharmacol* 26(3):130-40, 2011.
7. Haack S, Seeringer A, Thürmann PA, Becker T, Kirchheiner J. Sex-specific differences in side effects of psychotropic drugs: genes or gender? *Pharmacogenomics* 10(9):1511-26, 2009.
8. Labbate LA. Psychotropics and sexual dysfunction: the evidence and treatments. *Adv Psychosom Med* 29:107-30, 2008.
9. Costa AM, Lima MS, Mari Jde J. A systematic review on clinical management of antipsychotic-induced sexual dysfunction in schizophrenia. *Sao Paulo Med J* 124(5):291-7, 2006.
10. Berner MM, Hagen M, Kriston I. Management of sexual dysfunction due to antipsychotic drug therapy. 2012 Update of *Cochrane Database Syst Rev,* Jan 24;(1):CD003546, 2007.
11. Stimmel GL, Gutierrez MA. Sexual dysfunction and psychotropic medications. *CNS Spectr* 11(8 Suppl 9):24-30, 2006.

12. Muscatello MR, Bruno A, Pandolfo G, Micò U, Settineri S, Zoccali R. Emerging treatments in the management of schizophrenia - focus on sertindole. *Drug Des Devel Ther* 7;4:187-201, 2010.
13. Montejo AL, Majadas S, Rico-Villademoros F, Llorca G, De La Gándara J, Franco M, Martín-Carrasco M, Aguera L, Prieto N; Spanish Working Group for the Study of Psychotropic-Related Sexual Dysfunction. Frequency of sexual dysfunction in patients with a psychotic disorder receiving antipsychotics. *J Sex Med* 7(10):3404-13, 2010.
14. Martin-Du PR, Baumann P. Sexual dysfunctions induced by antidepressants and antipsychotics. *Rev Med Suisse* 26;4(150):758-62, 2008.
15. Pope A, Adams C, Paton C, Weaver T, Barnes TR. Assessment of adverse effects in clinical studies of antipsychotic medication: survey of methods used. *Br J Psychiatry*. 197(1):67-72, 2010.
16. Hanssens L, L'Italien G, Loze JY, Marcus RN, Pans M, Kerselaers W. The effect of antipsychotic medication on sexual function and serum prolactin levels in community-treated schizophrenic patients: results from the Schizophrenia Trial of Aripiprazole (STAR) study (NCT00237913). *BMC Psychiatry*. 2008 Dec 22;8:95, 2008.
17. Serretti A, Chiesa A. Sexual side effects of pharmacological treatment of psychiatric diseases. *Clin Pharmacol Ther* 89(1):142-7, 2011.
18. Drugs@FDA.gov labeling
19. Schöttle D, Kammerahl D, Huber J, Briken P, Lambert M, Huber CG. Sexual problems in patients with schizophrenia. *Psychiatr Prax* 36(4):160-8, 2009.

Chapter 14

1. Sherins R J, DeVita VT, Jr. Effect of drug treatment for lymphoma on male reproductive capacity. Studies of men in remission after therapy. *Ann Intern Med* 79:216-20, 1973.
2. Siris ES, Leventhaln BG, Vaitukaitis J. Effects of childhood leukemia and chemotherapy on puberty and reproductive function in girls. *New Engl J Med* 294:1143-46, 1976.
3. Witjes FJ, Debruyne FM, Fernandez del Moral P, Geboers AD. Ketoconazole high dose in management of hormonally pretreated patients with progressive metastatic prostate cancer. Dutch South-Eastern Urological Cooperative Group. *Urology* 33 (5):411, 1989.
4. Eil C. Ketoconazole binds to the human androgen receptor. *Horm Metab Res* 24 (8):367–70, 1992.
5. McHaffie DJ, Guz A, Johnston A. Impotence in patients on disopyramide. *Lancet, p 859*, 16 Apr, 1977.
6. Van Thiel DH, Gavaler JS, Smith WI et al. Hypothalamic-pituitary-gonadal dysfunction in men using cimetidine. *New Engl J Med* 300:1012-15, 1979.

Chapter 15

1. Inglewood EH Jr, Rockwell WJK. Effect of drug use on sexual behavior. *Med Aspects Hum Sex* 9:10-32, 1975.

2. Hollister LE. Drugs and sex and behavior in man. *Psychopharmacol Bull* 11:44, 1975.
3. Nail RL, Gunderson EF, Kolb D. Motives for drug use among light and heavy users. *J Nerv Ment Dis* 159:131-36, 1974.
4. Gay GR, Newmeyer JA, Elion RA, et al. Drug/sex practice in the Haight-Ashbury or "the sensuous hippie." Proc 37th Annual Scientific Meeting Committee on Problems of Drug Dependence. Washington, D.C. May 19-21, 1975, pp 1080-1101.
5. Gay GR, Sheppard CW. Sex in the "drug culture." *Med Aspects Hum Sex* 6:28-50, 1972.
6. Bush PJ. *Drugs, Alcohol & Sex*. New York: Marek, 1980.
7. Wells B. *Psychedelic Drugs*. Baltimore: Penguin Books, 1974.
8. Goode E. *The Marijuana Smokers*. New York: Basic Books, 1970.
9. Tart CT. *On Being Stoned. A Psychological Study of Marijuana Intoxication*. Palo Alto, Calif.: Science and Behavior Books, 1971.
10. Gay GR, Newmeyer JA, Elion, RA, et al. Drug/sex practice in the Haight-Ashbury or "the sensuous hippie." Proc 37th Annual Scientific Meeting Committee on Problems of Drug Dependence. Washington, D.C., May 19-21, 1975.
11. Gay GR, Sheppard CW. Sex in the "drug culture." *Med Aspects Hum Sex* 6:28-50, 1972.
12. Snyder SH. *Uses of Marijuana*. New York: Oxford University Press, 1971
13. Parr D. Sexual aspects of drug abuse in narcotic addicts. *Brit J Addict* 71:261-68, 1976.
14. Piemme TE. Sex and illicit drugs. *Med Aspects Hum Sex* 10:85-86, 1976.
15. DeLeon G, Wexler HK. Heroin addiction: its relation to sexual behavior and sexual experience. *J Abnormal Psychol* 81:36-38, 1973.
16. Mills LC. Drug-induced impotence. *Amer Fam Phys* 12:104-6, 1975.
17. Gossop MR. Addiction to narcotics: a brief review of the "junkie" literature. *Brit J Addict* 71:192-95, 1976.
18. Weir JG. The pregnant narcotic addict: a psychiatrist's impression. *Proc R. Soc Med* 65:869-70, 1972.
19. Burroughs W. *Junkie*. New York: Ace Books, 1953.
20. Cocteau J. *Opium: The Diary of a Cure*. London: New English Library, 1972.
21. Lowry TP. The volatile nitrites as sexual drugs: a user survey. *J Sex Educ Therap* 1:8-10, 1979.
22. Everett G. Amyl nitrite ("poppers") as an aphrodisiac. In Sandier M & Gessa G L (eds) *Sexual Behavior—Pharmacology and Biochemistry*. New York: Raven Press, 1975
23. Lange WR, Haertzen CA, Hickey JL, et al. Nitrite inhalants patterns of abuse in Baltimore and Washington, D.C. *Am J Drug Abuse* 14:29-39, 1988.
24. Sjovist F, Garle M, Rane A. Use of doping agents, in particular anabolic steroids, in sports and society. *Lancet* 371:1872, 2008
25. Hildebrandt T, Harty S, Langenbucher JW. Fitness supplements as a gateway substance for anabolic-androgenic steroid use. *Psychol Addict Behav* 26:955-62, 2012.
26. Calfee R, Fadale P. Popular ergogenic drugs and supplements in young atheletes. *Pediatrics* 117:577-89, 2006.
27. Goldman B, Bush P, Klatz R. *Death in the Locker Room*. Tucson, AZ: The Body Press, pp 89-90, 1987.

CPSIA information can be obtained at www.ICGtesting.com
Printed in the USA
BVOW06s1914030316

438981BV00015B/189/P

9 781478 738404